The Electric Corset
and Other Victorian Miracles

T0197963

The Electric Corset and Other Victorian Miracles

Medical Devices and Treatments from the Golden Age of Quackery

JEREMY AGNEW

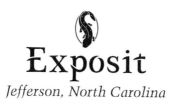

Exposit

Jefferson, North Carolina

ISBN (print) 978-1-4766-8383-6
ISBN (ebook) 978-1-4766-4526-1

LIBRARY OF CONGRESS AND BRITISH LIBRARY
CATALOGUING DATA ARE AVAILABLE

Front cover image: Advertising leaflet. The corset was recommended
for "all ladies suffering from any bodily ailment ... they perform
astonishing cures and invigorate every part of the system," London,
Pall Mall Electric Association, 1882, "The Pall Mall Electric Association,
Limited, 21, Holborn Viaduct, London, E.C." (Welcome Collection)

Printed in the United States of America

Exposit is an imprint of McFarland & Company, Inc., Publishers

Exposit

*Box 611, Jefferson, North Carolina 28640
www.expositbooks.com*

For Steve,
my business partner a long time ago,
who inadvertently involved us
in the world of medical humbug

Table of Contents

Preface

The practice of medicine is based on the prevention of disease, and the art and science of healing. The field of medicine has undergone constant change over the past two thousand years as new theories and techniques have been brought to bear on illness, thus medicine has been influenced by the particular culture, time, and place in which it has been practiced.

Treating the sick and injured has been a part of medicine since before recorded history, and devices to assist in treatment gradually evolved as a part of medical practice. Some of the first "medical devices" were amulets and talismans used by the earliest healers to assist them in the treatment process. Later, Roman and Greek physicians developed various medical instruments and appliances to support their healing efforts. Specialized knives, for example, were developed for use in their primitive surgery, needles and thread were used for closing wounds, and forceps were improved to assist with treating injuries and performing operations. Specialized drills were developed for cutting holes in the skull to treat brain injuries and headaches and, with misguided zeal, in an attempt to allow evil spirits that were thought to cause madness to escape from the inside of the head. Foreshadowing modern physical therapy, the Greek physician Galen developed a technique for treating disorders of the spine with a device that stretched the patient out flat on an apparatus with pulleys and ropes attached to the arms and legs, even though its use looked somewhat like a rack used for medieval torture.

Gradually, scientific medical instruments and devices were developed to assist in the diagnostic process, including various types of speculums to allow internal visualization of body cavities, the stethoscope to

1

listen to sounds of the heart, and the ophthalmoscope to diagnose the condition of blood vessels at the back of a patient's eye.

Scientific advances during the age of enlightenment included new developments in medicine and a better understanding of the human body. However, as the 1800s dawned, patients started to realize that the standard methods of bleeding and purging that had been the primary methods of treatment for hundreds of years were not generally effective and were certainly unpleasant. The public was ready for less invasive, less painful, alternative methods of healing. Even established physicians started to question the effectiveness of the old methods.

The early Victorian era of the mid–1800s saw the rise of various alternative medical movements, such as homeopathy, naturopathy, hydropathy, Thomsonian medicine, phrenology, mesmerism, and spiritualism. The time was right for these healers who promoted themselves and their treatments as painless and easy. Each of the new methods was a break from the traditional medicine of the time and each claimed to use more natural methods of healing. But along with the legitimate healers came medical quacks who capitalized on the realization that many of the Americans who wanted inexpensive, painless, easy-to-use cures for use in the privacy of their own homes could be a golden source of revenue.

The last half of the nineteenth century and the first few decades of the twentieth form a fascinating, yet somewhat perplexing, time in the history of medicine. This period formed the transition between ancient and modern medicine, between the antiquated treatments of bleeding and purging, and advances in better understanding disease processes and causes, and various medical treatments that formed the basis for moving into the modern age of scientific medicine.

As new scientific phenomena emerged in the 1800s to help explain the world around us, new forms of energy were discovered. One result was that these new discoveries, including electricity, magnetism, X-rays, and radioactivity, were quickly applied to the healing arts.

These mysterious unseen forces of radiant energy were quickly theorized to relate to the basic energy of the body itself. Radiant energy, which travels via wave motion, extends over a wide spectrum of frequencies. At the low end of the energy spectrum are sound waves that are audible to the human ear. At the upper end are cosmic rays that travel to (and through) our bodies from outer space. In between are other types of energy, including the visible spectrum of light that we observe with our eyes and X-rays that are powerful enough to penetrate the human body. By the end of the nineteenth century and early in the twentieth, different types of energy from across the spectrum were being applied to the human body in the hopes of finding new ways to treat and cure illness. An appendix at the back of this book outlines the radiant energy spectrum in ascending order of frequency to help place these forms of energy in perspective.

The late Victorian time period coincided with the national emergence of the widespread application of electricity. Electricity was seen as a new wonder source of mysterious energy and, like radioactivity several decades later, was seen as a modern scientific method to replenish the body's energy and to effect cures for a variety of diseases. As a result, electrical medical devices proliferated, some medically useful, some questionable, and some downright fraudulent.

The following chapters will look at some of the peculiar medical devices and treatments that emerged from the new health movement and which were promoted for use in assisting the cure of illnesses. Because of the explosion of new technology during the 1800s and early 1900s, the text will necessarily focus primarily on this time period, when the most bogus devices were developed and used. That was the era when new science, new technology, and new inventions converged to apply to all areas of life, including medical treatments. Many of these new medical devices used crude therapies based on simplistic ideas and theories. Some were developed from as simple a concept that if a patient recovered after a certain treatment, then the cure was the result of the treatment, no matter how outlandish it was. The following pages will describe some of the seemingly odd devices and cures that were developed by both legitimate physicians and fraudulent ones to assist in treating patients.

This book, however, is not a simple listing of some of the odd and peculiar medical devices that have been used to treat the human body. The text also focuses on the background of these treatments and devices. As well as descriptions of the devices themselves, this book takes a broader view of unorthodox medical appliances and discusses the medical rationale and practices of the time that led to their use.

Though correctly speaking the term "Victorian" refers to the time period between 1837 and 1901, when the English monarch Victoria was on the throne, the description "Victorian" will also be used in this book in a broader sense to designate the characteristic moral and social climate that existed in Great Britain and the United States during the last half of the nineteenth century. This was the time when medicine underwent a change from the early humoral theories of the Greek physician Galen to a more scientifically-based type of medical care. But, not without cause, this era has also been called the Golden Age of Quackery.

The reader will note, as a recurrent theme, the obsession of medical practitioners with treating the bowels. The concept, which was rooted in Egyptian and Greek medicine, was prominent through the eighteenth and nineteenth centuries as a generic form of treatment intended to expel disease by forcing the bowels to action, often in a violent manner. The idea soared to new heights in the eighteenth century, and was inherited by the Victorians. This obsession was continued into the medical concept of autointoxication that was extremely popular in the last two decades of the 1800s and the first three of the 1900s, and the idea that people were being poisoned from within by their own natural bodily processes.

It should be noted that this book is not a discussion of patent medicines or quack cures using drugs. Though the subject of patent medicines is closely tied to quack medicine and bogus practitioners, and patent medicines did form a large part of questionable medical practices from about the 1870s to 1930, that is not the focus of this book. Patent medicines have been described in detail in other books. The following chapters will focus on some of the peculiar devices and treatments used by both fringe and legitimate healers, and will place them in the context of contemporary medicine.

The discussion will also try to present a balanced perspective on what was and what was not legitimate treatment. Promoters of some of these peculiar devices and treatments were not all frauds and quacks, but some were legitimate and respectable physicians who believed that they were doing the best they could for their patients. Some of the treatments described may appear ludicrous to us now and, from our perspective, even barbaric. But, no matter how odd the treatments, many of them reflected the beliefs and knowledge of medical science of an earlier age. Physicians in the 1850s looked back on much of Roman medicine as being odd and incorporating strange remedies. By the same token, much of today's medicine will probably seem primitive to doctors of the future.

Most physicians genuinely believed in and practiced the latest discoveries in medicine, even if they later turned out to be less than useful. Thus, the application of what might today be considered odd and peculiar to us, or even quack treatment, was not always deception, but was the use of what current medical opinion believed to be the best treatment method at the time. In the late 1700s, for example, eminent physician Benjamin Rush from Philadelphia firmly believed in bleeding patients for illness and that, by doing so, he was performing the appropriate and best treatment for them.

The important concept here is that physicians worked with the latest medical knowledge of their time. It is difficult, therefore, to arbitrarily categorize many of the devices described in this book as quack devices, because some were legitimately used as the acceptable treatments of the time. Indeed, many of the questionable practitioners were as concerned about treating ailments correctly as were regular practitioners. From this perspective then, the term quackery should be defined not as ineffective therapy, but should rather emphasize fraudulent intent on the part of the promoter and practitioner. The word denotes not so much ignorance as it does dishonesty and deception.

Though many of the devices described in this book have later been categorized as "quack" medical devices, many of them, such as electrotherapy devices, were developed and used by the leading legitimate medical practitioners of the day. This was not quackery, but was considered to be the latest in medical technology. More in the questionable category would be devices like the Pillow Inhaler, which was a pillow filled with medicines that were said to destroy germs while the user slept. Quackery often becomes categorized only with hindsight.

Another part of the story is the creation of the U.S. Food and Drug Administration regulations, which were initially developed to control the labeling of food and patent medicines, and eventually to regulate medical devices. Until 1976 and the passage of the modern Medical Devices Amendment to the 1938 Food, Drug, and Cosmetic Act, there was very little legal control of fraudulent or ineffective medical devices.

The original Food and Drug Act of 1906 was concerned with the fraudulent labeling of food and medicines, and did not extend to quack medical devices. At the time, fraudulent medical devices had to be prosecuted in roundabout ways under existing postal laws and federal food and drug labeling laws. Thus it was easy for quacks to develop, promote, and sell a bogus medical device without much fear of any particular legal consequences. This, and its implications, will also be discussed in further detail.

So, armed with this background, let us venture into the shadowy world of quack healers and some of their peculiar devices, their often even more peculiar medical theories, and their bogus medical equipment. This is the world where healing through magnetizing the blood, electric baths to drive heavy metals from the body, electrical shocks to the genitals from battery-powered belts, and drinking radioactive water were trumpeted as successful, scientific, and modern alternatives to the conventional medical treatments of the time.

But, as we shall see, let the consumer beware!

ONE

Time for a Change

This book is a history of some of the peculiar, and often fraudulent, medical devices and practices that have been used to treat human ailments. In particular, the primary concentration will be on those devices that emerged in the 1800s and early 1900s. The largest growth of technological devices to treat human ailments occurred during this period as a result of several converging factors.

As an outgrowth of the explosion of patent medicines during the last part of the nineteenth century and early twentieth, there was a rapid rise in the number of health practitioners who promoted questionable medical devices. This should not be unexpected as it was the beginning of the age of mechanisms. This was the time of the introduction of technology into the home, such as the electric light, the radio, electric household appliances, and the automobile. So it is not without basis that the late nineteenth century and early twentieth century was the high point of the historical era of medical quackery.[1]

Another element in the story was the changing state of medicine due to new theories and a more scientific understanding of the disease process. However, the specialized diagnostic equipment that is commonly used today did not exist until well into the twentieth century. The doctor went to the patient, not the patient to a well-equipped clinic. Doctors, particularly in rural areas, made house calls either by horse, wagon, or horse-and-buggy, with their surgical kit and drugs stowed with them. Many practiced out of their saddlebags, and carried their meager supplies with them to the patient in an old-time doctor's black bag.

The medical equipment on these visits consisted of a kit that contained everything that the doctor might need to treat illness, deliver a child, or perform minor surgery. The doctor's black bag typically contained various knives for surgery, a lancet for performing bleeding, probes for exploring and dilating body canals, forceps for clamping bleeding veins and arteries, scissors, tweezers, needle and thread for sewing up wounds, obstetrical instruments for childbirth, and a bone saw for amputating limbs and extremities.

The doctor's bag also carried bottles of medicine so that the physician could immediately dispense the appropriate drugs during his visit. Common medicines were emetics, such as ipecac and mustard, and purgatives, such as calomel, castor oil, jalap, and senna. A small amount of quinine might be included for treating malaria.

Medical Education

The rise in popularity of various types of peculiar medical devices that grew and flourished during this period had its roots in a mistrust by the general public of nineteenth-century physicians and the medicine they practiced. Two important factors contributed to the problem. One was the state of medical education. The other was the methods of treatment that physicians employed.

The first factor: Most physicians in the 1700s had only a rudimentary education, and a lack of formal credentials often created a distrust among the public. Few doctors had much formal medical training and many of them called themselves "doctor" simply because they took care of patients. Most colonial physicians supplemented their income by having another business to fall back on, such as farming or owning an apothecary shop. There were no licensing authorities, no medical schools, no hospitals, no medical reference literature, and no regulations on doctors.

As there was a widespread lack of medical schools in America, there were few university-educated physicians in the country. When the Revolutionary War started in 1775, only approximately 10 percent of the doctors practicing in the original thirteen colonies had a medical degree that resulted from formal training; the rest had been trained by the apprentice system. The first medical school in America was at the College of Philadelphia, opened in 1765.

Even by the nineteenth century, the amount and quality of medical education was highly variable and often inadequate. At the time the frontier was pushing west towards California in the 1840s, there were no medical schools west of the Mississippi. Doctors with medical degrees from institutions of higher learning in the East were few and, even then, the quality of training received by doctors varied tremendously. Students were often accepted to medical school without any formal education. In 1870 Harvard Medical School gave no written exams because most of the students could not write well enough.

There were two primary pathways to becoming a doctor in the mid–1800s. One of them was to attend one of the few medical schools that were available in the United States (in 1830 there were 22). Another option for those with enough money was to study in Europe, though this was not an easy route. Oxford and Cambridge universities in England granted medical degrees, but required 14 years of study and that the student belong to the Church of England. Another possibility, though expensive, was to attend the Royal College of Physicians in Edinburgh, Scotland, which was probably the best medical school in Europe in the second half of the eighteenth century. Other important medical schools were in Paris, London, and Leyden, Netherlands.

The bigger problem for hopeful medical students in America was that few of them had the financial resources to study in Europe, so the common pathway to becoming a physician was through another option, the apprentice system. In this method, potential doctors served an apprenticeship under a practicing physician. The teaching method was primarily hands-on training and the observation of cases. This option took anywhere from one to seven years to complete, with the average time being about three years.

There were arguments to be made for both methods. Physicians who graduated from formal university training typically gained more knowledge from books and had a better understanding of medical theory. On the other hand, doctors who qualified under the apprentice system generally had more hands-on experience. Whichever method of training was used, the rate of cures was poor because there was little understanding of the disease process. Interestingly, the original meaning of the word "cure" meant only to care for the ill, and did not have the modern meaning of a treatment that is successfully applied to individuals to restore them to health.

Before 1840, only a third of the practicing doctors in New England had attended a medical school or completed an apprenticeship.[2] Lax standards for medical licensing allowed some medical diplomas to be awarded after a six-month correspondence course.[3] Many quacks and pretenders simply displayed fake medical certificates or went by titles that they had conferred on themselves.[4] It was not until the 1880s and 1890s that most states adopted licensing requirements for physicians.[5]

Humoral Medicine

The second problem that created a distrust of doctors was that even by the early 1800s medical science had made few advances beyond the humoral theories that formed the basis of Hippocratic medicine taught to physicians in ancient Greece.

Roman and Greek medicine had their roots in Egyptian medicine. Humoral medicine was further formalized in the teachings of the Greek physician Hippocrates in the late fifth century BC. His theories were further refined 700 years later in the second century AD with the theories of the Greek physician and writer Galen. This still formed the basis of medical practice in the early 1800s.

Galen taught that the body was ruled by four bodily fluids, called humors, which determined a person's personality and reaction to disease. These fluids were blood (*sanguis*), phlegm (*pituita*), yellow bile (*chole*), and black bile (*melanchole*), which originated in the heart, brain, liver, and spleen respectively. Each humor was associated with one of the four seasons of the year and its qualities corresponded to the four earthly elements of air, water, fire, and earth. The humors also combined the fundamental qualities of warm, cold, wet, and dry. Blood, for example, was thought to make the body warm and wet, and yellow bile warm and dry, while phlegm was considered make it cold and wet, and black bile cold and dry.

The manner in which the humors were combined was thought to be responsible for every individual's bodily characteristics, such as weight, personality, and even the amount of body hair. Blood had the quality of heat, which was thought to produce a fiery personality. Phlegm was moist and produced a calm personality. Yellow bile was cold and made a person bad-tempered. Black bile was dry and resulted in a personality that was melancholic. The colors of the humors were also theorized to be combined to produce the hue of people's skin and made different people red, white, or yellow, and swarthy or pale.

The fundamental theory of Greek and Roman medicine was that health was a state of harmony of bodily processes and humors. Thus, while good health was due to a stable equilibrium of the humors, illness and disease were caused by an imbalance.

As a result of the continuation of these theories through the ages, the practice of medicine during the first half of the nineteenth century was still in a primitive state. Scientifically valid medical knowledge was limited in scope, and physicians did not yet understand the role of bacteria in causing disease. A diagnosis of disease might be as vague and nebulous as "inflammation of the chest," "malignant bilious fever," "catarrh of the liver," or simply "the jim-jams" (*delirium tremens* due to acute alcoholism).

As time went on, the diagnosis of different diseases improved, but the treatments for them did not. Even though diseases gradually became better recognized and differentiated, physicians could typically only treat the patient's symptoms rather than using a scientific cure to attack the cause of the disease.

Unable to see inside the body or to scientifically analyze blood or other internal body fluids, physicians used observation of the products of the body as their primary diagnostic tool. The release of noxious material from the body of someone who was ill through vomiting, sweating, urination, and diarrhea was seen as evidence of the body ridding itself of troublesome and putrid material that was causing the disease.

The Dreaded Cures

Because disease was considered to be an imbalance in the humors, the reasoning followed that the cure for illness was to bring the humors back into balance. The extension of this thinking was that if the vomiting, sweating, urination, and defecation that accompanied disease could be forced to occur, then the doctor would be putting the patient back on the road to health. Medical practice, therefore, based "cures" for disease on removing the excess of troublesome humors or any impure substances by forcibly expelling them from the body.

Expelling disease from the body was a common medical practice. One method used in ancient times was with the use of the aptly-named plant sneezeweed (*Helenium autumnale*) from the daisy family. The dried leaves were crushed and used to make snuff. When inhaled, the powder induced sneezing, which supposedly blew evil spirits, including those that caused disease, out of the body.

To accomplish the goal of forcibly expelling the troublesome products of illness from the body, patients were more commonly subjected to a series of violent treatments that involved bleeding, purging, blistering, vomiting, and sweating. From about the sixth century to the sixteenth, medical treatments to achieve this were carried out by medical specialists. At the top of the profession were the physicians, both the elite at the summit of the medical pyramid who were trained at a university that awarded an academic degree, and the lower ones who were trained through an apprentice program. Physicians, however, only prescribed drugs. They received their name from "physic," which was a name for medicines, particularly cathartics (often called "physicking pills"), so their traditional therapies consisted mostly of various ways to make the bowels work vigorously.

Next below the physicians in ranking were the barber-surgeons, who treated everything that could not be treated by prescribing drugs. Barbers had razors for shaving clients and thus were considered to be the ideal candidates for any care of the body that required cutting, from cutting hair to cutting off damaged limbs. Barber-surgeons were the most common medical practitioners of the Middle Ages, and were happy to carry out medical procedures to supplement their income from shaving faces and cutting hair.

After about the eleventh century, the physical side of medicine, such as bleeding, surgery, the treatment of external injuries, amputations, pulling teeth, removing calluses, setting broken bones, administering clysters, dressing wounds, and other physical manipulation of the body, were transferred almost exclusively to barber-surgeons. Bleeding,

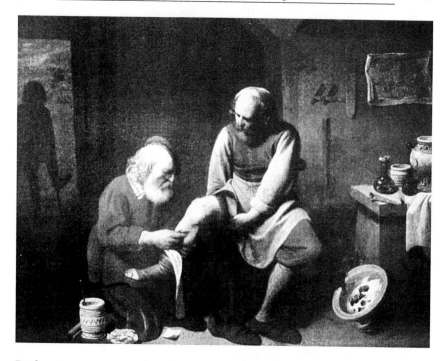

Barber-surgeons were the most common medical practitioners of the Middle Ages, performing care for all types of medical problems that were not treated by prescribing drugs. Barbers used razors for surgery from bloodletting to amputating damaged limbs. This painting by David Ryckært from the 1600s shows a village barber-surgeon bleeding a vein in a patient's leg. Draining blood from a patient to cure illness by supposedly re-balancing the humors was a concept that originated in Roman and Greek medicine (National Library of Medicine).

in particular, was a treatment that they performed. The classic barber pole of red, white, and blue spiral stripes is said to have been used to advertise this surgical side of their profession. The red stripe symbolized blood, the white symbolized the tourniquet or bandage used during bleeding, and the blue represented the vein that was bled.[6] In cruder displays, barbers in London in 1307 were criticized for advertising their services by displaying buckets of blood and bloody rags outside their establishments.[7]

By the 1700s the two professions of the barber-surgeon parted. Barbers returned to tending to hair and beards, and surgeons became part of a legitimate specialized field that provided most of the hands-on part of medical care. Surgeons learned their trade by apprenticeship and were regulated by guilds, though the division of labor was not totally clear-cut because physicians also occasionally performed some physical treatments.[8]

Only a few surgeons attempted to perform complicated operations, though remarkably they performed the surgical removal of bladder stones. The pain from a stone was usually so intense that patients were willing to accept surgery without the benefit of anesthesia (luckily for the patient in as little as 45 seconds if the surgeon was skilled) and accepted the near-certain risk of infection, even though they knew that the mortality rate for this particular operation was about 50 percent.[9]

The lowest category of the medical ranks was the apothecary, who filled out physicians' prescriptions for medicine and did the menial medical work that physicians and surgeons did not want to do, such as administering clysters. Apothecaries were trained through an apprentice system that lasted from five to seven years, mostly involving observation and hands-on training. They then sought admittance to a guild in order to obtain a license to practice.

Heroic Medicine

The aim of medical providers was to rid the body of infections and illness by removing excess blood from the body, flushing out the intestines by purging and vomiting, and inducing sweat to perspire out toxins. Purging and vomiting were particularly favored as they treated both ends of the intestinal tract to remove supposed disease-causing "impurities." These violent remedies were the collective cornerstones of "Heroic Medicine," a type of treatment for disease that originated in Europe and found its way to the United States. The classic era of Heroic Medicine in America ran from roughly 1780 to 1850.

These treatments, however, were not without side effects that often caused further distress for the patient. Bleeding created a serious drop in blood pressure, and made patients weak and anemic. Purging caused a loss of vital bodily fluids and electrolytes, and often eventually poisoned the patient with mercury from the drug calomel that was commonly used. Blistering created skin damage and produced open patches of flesh that could easily become infected.

An excess of blood was blamed for many illnesses, including the fevers that arose from infectious diseases, and the use of bleeding was believed to be a cure for almost every known ailment. Bleeding was thought to reduce the inflammation that accompanied many diseases and to restore balance to the body. An overabundance of blood was also blamed for "morbid excitement" and irritability in a patient. Bleeding was *the* preferred treatment and was used to treat everything from epilepsy to bruises.

One of the champions of bleeding was Benjamin Rush, an eminent American physician who studied medicine at the Royal College of Physicians in Edinburgh and the College of New Jersey in Philadelphia. He was one of the most influential physicians in America at the time and is generally considered to be the father of American medicine. Rush argued that the cause of sickness was congested arteries and veins that could only be relieved by the removal of blood. When Rush was taken ill in 1813 and subsequently weakened, he demanded that he be bled. He insisted on the treatments, and repeated bleedings probably hastened his own death.[10]

Bleeding was accomplished by cutting open a small vein and allowing some of the patient's blood to drain out. The incision was typically placed near the site of pain or illness. For example, bleeding a vein under the tongue or in the neck was used to treat inflammation in the throat or for problems involving the ear. Bleeding was even applied to veins in such sensitive areas as hemorrhoids or in the penis.

Cutting was accomplished by using either a lancet (a sharp surgical knife, also called a fleam) or a scarificator, which was a metal box with a series of spring-loaded sharp knife-like steel blades that created cuts in the skin. Another method was to apply leeches to the affected area and let them suck the blood out.

The only variations in bleeding treatments were: when they should be performed, the location, how often they should be performed, and how much blood should be withdrawn. A typical bleeding treatment removed a pint or more of blood, which was continued if there was no apparent improvement. If symptoms did not subsequently subside, the bleeding was repeated.

Another of the essential treatments of Heroic Medicine was purging the intestinal tract by various processes in order to supposedly expel the cause of the disease and re-balance the humors. Cleansing the bowels to drive out "impure" humors was accomplished by using a series of purgative drugs, or clysters. Periodic purging of a patient, even when not ill, was also thought to promote general good health through purity of the bowels, because neglect of the bowels was thought to send a person down the pathway to appalling disease. Just as the loss of blood created by extensive bleeding calmed the patient due to exhaustion, so did violent purging of the bowels. Therefore, to some extent, blood-letting and purging did suppress the symptoms of diseases, though obviously not the causes.

Another popular method for trying to restore the balance of the humors by ridding the body of supposed substances that caused disease was to have the patient vomit them out. The use of an emetic drug was intended to expel supposed disease-causing humors through the upper end of the internal tract by inducing violent vomiting. The theory was that the ejection of the stomach contents would remove the toxic material that was causing the illness.

A fourth popular treatment, often used in conjunction with bleeding, purging, and vomiting in Heroic Medicine, was to rid the body of noxious poisons and bad humors by forcing them to escape through the skin by sweating. The underlying theory was that if the pores of the skin were clogged, waste matter was trapped inside the body where it would poison the individual from the inside, and thus needed to be driven out in the form of heavy perspiration.

Another method, similar to sweating, to drive bad humors out through the skin was blistering. This was accomplished by applying various irritating chemicals to the skin that caused large blisters to form. The theory was that this procedure drew out any internal inflammation by bringing poisonous products to the surface of the skin and collecting them in the form of these large blisters, thus sucking the "bad" humors from the body.

These standard treatments for illness were antiquated and unpleasant. Patients disliked them and found them to be physically debilitating. And they developed a fear of them because many patients died anyway after these treatments. The role of bacteria in disease was as yet unknown, so in cases of severe gastrointestinal infections, such as cholera or typhoid, the disease's resulting vomiting, cramps, and diarrhea, exacerbated by a physician's bleeding, and induced vomiting and purging which unbalanced the body's electrolyte levels, often resulted in the patient's dying from dehydration.[11]

As a result, the public started to question the nature of proper and appropriate medical treatment, the role of physicians in American society, and the definition of good health. People who became ill tried to find alternatives to these brutal "cures," in the hopes of finding gentler and safer treatments.

The Decline of Heroic Medicine

Medicine changed dramatically from the early seventeenth century to the turn of the twentieth, assisted by the rise of scientific methodology and tools as scientists and physicians worked to find new methods of treatment based on new medical discoveries.

In the colonial period there was no real expectation that medical treatment would cure illness, because medicine had little in the way of true therapeutic cures. Health care providers did not understand the causes of diseases and were therefore unable to offer reliable remedies. Surgery was primarily limited to amputation of damaged extremities, sewing up cuts, and splinting minor cases of broken bones.

Most medical "discoveries" were based on speculative theories. In all fairness, this was due to a lack of knowledge, and not the fault of physicians, as they did not have a proper understanding of the disease process, particularly the role of germs. For example, cures that were recommended during epidemics included plugging the nostrils with tobacco leaves, lighting fires outside to burn away bad air, and firing cannons and muskets into the air to break up the "diseased atmosphere."[12]

Few therapies were effective for curing disease at the beginning of the nineteenth century, so Heroic Medicine continued to be the accepted course of treatment for illness during the late 1700s and first half of the 1800s. Due to the healing power of nature and the ability of the human body to cure itself, many patients actually recovered in spite of these treatments, which led physicians to believe that their treatments had been effective.

Patients expected doctors to perform successful cures all the time, some of which may have been impossible given the level of contemporary knowledge and technology. Any failure to achieve a satisfactory cure, however, whether the fault lay with the doctor or a patient too ill to be cured, resulted in a low level of confidence in doctors. In many cases this was a circular pathway. Much of the deep-rooted skepticism of doctors was caused by their limited success in curing illnesses, part of which may have been due to the fact that ill people did not go to doctors until it was too late to be cured. Treatment was sometimes delayed either because of the cost or because the nearest doctor was too far away. The high death rate, in turn, made sick people more reluctant to visit a doctor, which resulted in a vicious cycle that delayed treatment and resulted in a high rate of mortality.

By the same token, doctors sometimes promised more than they could deliver. However, the blame should not be totally placed on the doctor, because most illnesses were caused by infection or disease agents whose causes were unknown at the time. American physicians stressed the fever theory, which vaguely stated that disease was caused by excessive "irritation" or "morbid excitement." As medical research progressed, scientists and physicians continued to find out more about the body's structure and function, but developed little in the way of new treatments.

The result of all this was that the practice of medicine in America during the first half of the nineteenth century was not much different than that practiced by the ancient Greeks and Romans. Not much was cured by these treatments and they often caused more injury to the patient than good. Bleeding removed essential blood and purging with drugs containing toxic metals often caused poisoning.

By the early 1800s the volume of blood that was being removed during bleeding and the amounts of calomel administered for purging were increased in an attempt to better subdue the bodily excitement that was perceived to accompany disease. There was no discrimination as to the patient's age, gender, or condition. The more serious the disease, the more intense the treatment. Improvements were usually marginal and the outcome after treatment was still a high mortality rate.

Seeing this, patients feared doctors for their brutal treatments and debatable education, and became concerned about the drugs that doctors were concocting out of poisonous substances, such as mercury, arsenic, and antimony. People suffering from disease, seeing the results of bleeding, vomiting, and purging on other patients—such as weakness, possible lifelong debility due to mercury poisoning, and often death—were understandably not enthusiastic about having it done. As a result, patients started to question the entire concept of conventional Heroic Medicine. In the early 1800s even some physicians started to question the effectiveness and necessity for the bleeding that killed so many, and the large doses of calomel and opium that were being prescribed. By the 1850s bleeding was starting to lose its popularity and by 1860 it was rarely used by doctors in the eastern United States.[13]

The late 1800s were a time of major changes in medical practice from the old methods of bleed-and-purge to newer, more scientific understanding and methods. Researchers were making progress in categorizing and identifying diseases; however, there was still a distinct lack of understanding of the workings of the inside of the human body. Any type of surgery to explore or treat the insides, such as the gall bladder, appendix, and even hernias, was highly risky due to surgical infection from unclean conditions. Antiseptic techniques used during surgery would not be developed until the discoveries of Joseph Lister in the late 1860s. The second drawback for the patient was pain. Inhaled anesthetics to make surgery painless were not introduced until the 1840s. The first successful appendectomy was not performed until 1883.

To be a surgeon before about 1870 meant a job that primarily involved bloodletting. After becoming a doctor, many did not perform surgery except as a last resort, because they had not received the proper training to perform it. Few surgeons were brave enough or competent enough to explore the inner workings of the abdomen until the late 1880s and 1890s. Thus the only reasonable access to the inside of the body and treatments for anything internal were limited to access through its natural openings at either end of the gastrointestinal tract. Medicine could be administered through the top end and the mouth with pills and potions, and to the lower part via the anus and rectum with suppositories or enemas. Limited access to the bladder could be achieved through urethra. Women could additionally be treated via the vagina.

Though the use of bleeding as a cure generally went out of favor by the mid–1800s, the other types of treatment, such as purging, sweating, and blistering continued in slightly different, medically-approved, forms through the end of the century. Sweating was reinvented with various types of hot baths. Purging the intestinal tract was continued through the use of colonic hydrotherapy at health spas and, in the early 1900s, through the widespread use of laxative patent medicines. Though these "cures" had drastic effects, they were often what patients wanted and at least made them feel that some active form of treatment was being performed to cure their condition.

Even by 1900 patients under a doctor's care had only a 50 percent chance of faring better than if they and their diseases had been left alone. Infectious diseases, such as pneumonia, tuberculosis, diphtheria, smallpox, and dysentery were responsible for more than a third of all deaths, but doctors had little to use to cure them.[14] Thus the public became skeptical about the ability of the conventional medicine of the time to cure disease. Although physicians had started to recognize specific symptoms and diseases, the contemporary treatments of bleeding and purging were unable to prevent or effectively treat many of these illnesses. Patients found the constant use of purgatives and emetics to be unpleasant and disagreeable to say the least, and wanted gentler treatments. As a result, many people started to consider alternative treatments that produced less stress on the body, but which appeared to be as effective in healing illness.

By the 1820s the time was right for health reforms and the introduction of new ideas of curing, and for techniques that departed from toxic and unpleasant treatment methods and poisonous drugs. The search for cures that were not as drastic as those used by Heroic Medicine led to the development of several other systems of treatment that were collectively referred to under the general heading of "irregular" medicine, as opposed to that practiced by "regular" or conventional medical practitioners. During the early 1800s these practitioners of alternative medicine started to make claims of being safer and surer in their cures than regular physicians. As a consequence, the public started to abandon conventional physicians as their primary caregivers.

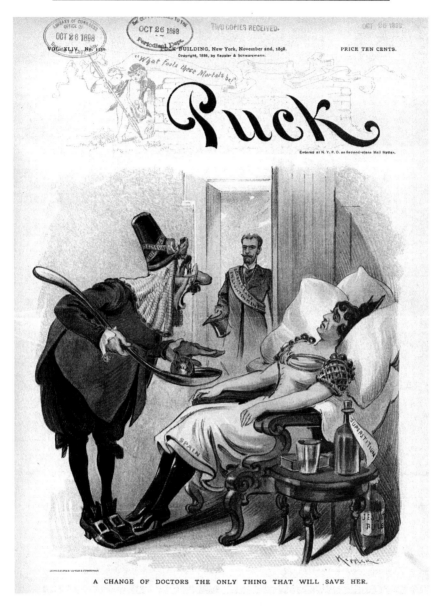

A CHANGE OF DOCTORS THE ONLY THING THAT WILL SAVE HER.

Though aimed at a contemporary political audience, this cartoon by Udo Keppler from *Puck* magazine in 1898 reflects the discontent with the old style of Heroic Medicine and the search for something new. The man labeled "Medieval Quack" is administering a large pill to a female figure reclining in a chair. The well-dressed man labeled "Science and Enlightenment," who is entering through the door in the background, symbolizes the desire for more effective and up-to-date medicine (Library of Congress).

The Rise of Alternative Medicine

Several methods of alternative medical treatment, such as the water-cure, homeopathy, botanical cures, osteopathy, and chiropractic, became popular during the first half of the nineteenth century. These methods were separate from regular medicine and were part of the movement away from conventional healing. Each methodology offered a cure through what their promoters felt were more natural healing methods, such as the use of pure water or medicinal herbs.

A distinction is usually drawn between what has been called orthodox, conventional, or mainstream medicine on one side and unconventional or "alternative medicine" on the other. In reality, there are not the two categories of conventional and alternative medicine. Instead, there are medical treatments that work and there are those that don't work. Whatever its origin, every treatment must be viewed on its own merits and must be tested objectively to determine whether it is or is not effective.

Three of the systems of alternative medicine that had the most impact were homeopathic medicine, botanical cures, and the water cure. Though their use generally encountered resistance from the conventional medical profession, all three methods of treatment grew in popularity between about 1830 and 1860.

The first treatment method that rivaled the established practice of medicine was homeopathy, which became a controversial, but popular, alternative to Heroic Medicine. Homeopathy was a non-painful alternative to bleeding and purging, and became one of the first significant medical systems that diverged from the conventional medicine of the time.

Homeopathic medicine used minute amounts of plant-based drugs for treatments. The concept originated in Germany around 1800 and flourished under the leadership of a German physician named Samuel Christian Hahnemann. Hahnemann's basic principle was what he called the "Law of Similars." He stated that a minute dose of a drug would cure disease in a sick person if the drug produced symptoms in a healthy person that were the same as the disease being treated. Hahnemann felt that the smaller the dosage of his homeopathic remedies, the more effective the cure. By the 1820s, homeopathic medicine had become very popular as part of the reaction against Heroic Medicine.

Homeopathy became popular in England and America in the 1840s and increased in popularity through the 1880s. For these forty or so years, homeopathy had a respectable enough following to challenge conventional medicine, but by the 1890s its popularity had started to decline.

The second important trend in the wave of alternative medical treatments was Thomsonianism and the medical use of botanical cures. Thomson's search for an alternative to Heroic Medicine began after his mother and wife suffered through illnesses during which they were given unpleasant heroic treatments.

Samuel A. Thomson was a New England farmer and self-taught practitioner who discovered through trial and error how certain herbs caused physical responses in sick people. As a result, Thomson developed a health movement that used plant-based therapies. In particular, Thomson claimed that most illnesses were due to an excess of cold in the body, so he and his practitioners treated their patients with hot baths and used plant-based remedies to induce perspiration. He theorized that if the body did not generate enough heat due to illness, he had to supply it from the outside.

Thomsonian treatments were claimed to be gentle and work with nature to support its activities, as opposed to attacking it with drugs. He maintained that disease resulted from a "clogging of the system," which was best alleviated by purging and sweating. The difference, however, was that he did not use bloodletting or treatment with toxic drugs to achieve these results, as did conventional physicians. He believed that remedies from plants were the only appropriate treatments; however, like the conventional physicians, Thomson still made the patient vomit to remove supposed impure substances, made them sweat to remove impurities through the skin, and administered clysters to cleanse the bowels. There were divided opinions on the effectiveness of Thomson's methods, but in actual fact, Thomson's remedies probably worked as well as anything else at the time.

Unfortunately, Thomson was one of the healers who fell into the common scientific trap of *post hoc* reasoning. He theorized that if a patient felt better after taking one of his herbal medicines, the plant must have cured the disease.

The third of the important new forms of gentler treatments was the water-cure championed by Vincent Preissnitz. He emphasized the novel idea at that time of using exercise and fresh air, accompanied by the use of large volumes of water to effect a cure, both externally with baths and internally through drinking. Preissnitz's water-cure system led directly to hydropathic cures and the later spas and sanatoriums where physicians recommended a variety of water treatments. Public disappointment with Heroic Medicine helped to make homeopathy and hydropathy very popular by the middle of the nineteenth century.[15]

Two of the other notable methods of alternative healing that became popular around the same time were osteopathy and chiropractic, both of which dealt with manipulation of the back and spine.

Osteopathy was developed after the American Civil War by physician and surgeon Andrew Taylor Still, who felt that the source of disease and imbalance in the body was due to misplaced bones of the spine. This system of alternative treatment involved the use of manual manipulation of the muscles and vertebrae of the back to cure disease by removing "obstructions inhibiting the flow of blood and nervous fluid."[16]

Chiropractic was another form of alternative medicine that involved diagnosis and treatment of the musculoskeletal system, particularly the spine. Chiropractic was developed by Daniel David Palmer, who believed, like Andrew Still, that misaligned vertebrae in the spine caused problems in the nervous system and were the origin of ill health. He reasoned that manipulation of the spine to bring the vertebrae back into correct alignment would resolve the problem. The name "chiropractic" was derived from Greek words meaning "done by hand."

For nine years Palmer followed a career as a magnetic healer, drawing his hands over a patient's body to draw out illness, before he changed to manipulating the vertebrae. Palmer felt that all illness was caused by skeletal subluxations and alleviating the subluxation cured the illness. A subluxation is a partial dislocation between the bones where some degree of contact is preserved between them. A full luxation occurs when a joint is dislocated and the bones are pulled apart.[17]

At the same time, the early 1800s saw the emergence of lay health reformers who viewed themselves as better interpreters of medical science than the conventional medical profession. These enthusiastic reformers saw declining health all around them that they thought could be corrected. They caught the attention of the public because their verbal attacks were part of a broader social analysis and critique of American culture as they worked to improve mankind to their own particular physical and moral standards. They combined righteousness and health into one topic, insisting that freedom from disease also included abstaining from any degenerate thoughts or habits, which included drinking, smoking, and too much attention to sex. Many health consumers did indeed feel these alternative treatments were preferable to the bleeding, purging, blistering, and sweating of conventional medicine.

The conventional medical view has been that alternative practitioners believed in absurd theories and sometimes dangerous therapies to treat serious conditions that could only be treated with scientific medicine. Even if these remedies were harmless, reputable physicians were concerned that patients might suffer and die because they did not receive the correct treatment for their condition, but were treated with random crude therapies based on simplistic theories. On the other hand, alternative practitioners considered themselves to be legitimate healers who were trying to cure without drugs and surgery.

Though the label of "quackery" has been applied to alternative or unorthodox medicine from its beginnings, some of these alternative cures were accepted and promoted by the conventional medical establishment. Many alternative practitioners wanted just as much as regular practitioners to heal sick people. The term quackery has historically been used less to denote ineffective therapy than to designate fraudulent intent on the part of the promoter. It is a category of medicine that describes not so much ignorance as dishonesty and deception.

The bottom line is that by the mid–1800s the time was right for people to look at alternative cures that offered treatments less dangerous and unpleasant than the regular medical profession was providing. The conditions were also right to create a ripe environment for quacks and frauds to spring forth with patent medicines and bizarre medical devices for the treatment of ailments.

But first a look at the tricksters and hucksters themselves.

Two

If It Quacks Like a Duck...

A history of medicine is generally the history of conventional orthodox treatments and qualified medical practitioners. However, woven into this is a series of peculiar treatments performed with peculiar medical devices and equipment. Unfortunately, persons with chronic or incurable illnesses have been sometimes abused by unscrupulous confidence men and swindlers who preyed on human fear and suffering as they peddled phony cures.

Medical historian Roy Porter has defined a quack as someone who operated outside of the definition of orthodox or regular medicine. The term was generally applied to a health practitioner who made extravagant claims for a product that did not work, or who had no legitimate medical science to support his claims. Quacks have often been associated with the patent medicine industry and salesmen who drummed up business through self-orchestrated publicity. These were individual entrepreneurs and businessmen who depended primarily on secret remedies rather than being part of the established medical community.[1]

Quackery

Quack is an abbreviation of the sixteenth-century Dutch term "quacksalver," which was the name for a person who sold salves and potions with a fast and noisy sales pitch that was said to sound like the quacking of a duck.[2] The lack of an effective cure after extravagant claims for various medicines led to them being categorized as "quack" medicines. The shortened name was eventually applied to fraudulent promoters of patent medicines and bogus "medical" devices, or as an adjective to describe the treatment or device itself. The name "quack" was used to describe an untrained person who practiced medicine fraudulently, claimed to be a physician but wasn't, or claimed to have medical knowledge that they really didn't. Another explanation is that "quacksalver" was a Dutch corruption of the word "quicksilver," one of the names for mercury, because mercury was widely used as a historical remedy to treat syphilis.[3]

There were several other names for fringe medical practitioners in Renaissance Europe. In medieval Italy, a performer who sold potions in public was known as a *mountebank* (Italian: *montimbanco*), because the salesman mounted a platform in a public place and attracted audiences by telling jokes and stories. Part of the pitch was pure showmanship with eye-catching costumes, colorful stage settings and scenery, music, the presence of exotic animals such as snakes and monkeys, and perhaps accomplices in the crowd to help persuade potential customers during the sales pitch.

Another Italian name for the itinerant salesmen who peddled patent medicines in public places was *ciarlatano*, which meant "to sell drugs in public places." The word later became the English word "charlatan" to describe a confidence man who knowingly sold quack medicines. The names mountebank, charlatan, and quack quickly took on derogatory connotations to describe an untrustworthy confidence man with a slick sales pitch who sold medicines that were not effective.[4]

The sales pitch from these medieval quacks usually sounded good, but was often incomprehensible. One German quack in the seventeenth century had the following to say about his patent medicine: "Gentlemen, I present you with my 'Universal Solvative,' which corrects all the Cacochymick and Cachexical Disease of the Intestines.... Secondly, My 'Friendly Pills' call'd the Never Failing Heliogenes, which by dilating and expanding the Gelastick Muscles, first of all discovered by myself. They clear the Officina Intelligentiae, correct the Exorbitancy of the Spleen, mundify the Hypogastrium, comfort the sphincter and are an excellent remedy against Propsero Chlorosis or green Sickness."[5] This convoluted pseudo-medical nonsense was very similar in obscurity to some of the sales pitches for questionable medical devices that appeared at the end of the nineteenth century. Quacks spouted enough pseudo-science to sound legitimate. This shameless method for promoting sales of patent medicines, and later by extension, quack medical devices, spread all over medieval Europe.

Patent Medicines

Long before complicated ineffective medical devices appeared, their counterparts in the drug world, quack patent medicines, were being sold through the mail and at medicine shows. In the late 1800s, uncertainty about the capability of doctors to cure diseases and the undesirability of undergoing bleeding and purging made the time right for patent medicines. Patent medicine sales were a pervasive and very profitable form of quackery.

Patent medicines, also called "proprietary medicines," were pills, tonics, and potions that were concocted by various manufacturers based on their own ideas of healing, and mostly without any curative powers. Few patent medicine manufacturers or sellers had any medical training. Patent medicines were not regulated and were freely available from any drugstore, from a medicine show salesman, or directly through the mail from the manufacturer. The medicine was often claimed to contain a secret ingredient known only to the manufacturer. The use of patent medicines started to flourish in the 1870s and peaked in the 1880s, though their popularity continued until the 1930s.

Most patent medicines claimed to offer cures for a long list of illnesses, including such diverse ailments as jaundice, dropsy, yellow fever, biliousness, tiredness, vertigo, flatulence, heartburn, kidney and liver diseases, cramps, vomiting, stomach distress, acid digestion, bloating, coughs, consumption, epilepsy, migraine, low blood pressure, high blood pressure, gallstones, strokes, bronchitis, whooping cough, and tuberculosis. In other words, almost everything. Cures for coughs, asthma, and consumption (tuberculosis) were popular in advertising because these diseases were so widespread.

One of the contemporary theories was that diseases arose from impurities in the blood, hence many patent medicines claimed that they would purify the blood. They also claimed that various impurities were trapped in the body and the medicines would purge them out, usually literally, as the user soon found out.

The use of patent medicines provided an alternative to the conventional drugs of the day. Instead of putting up with medical treatment that consisted primarily of the unpleasant routines of bleeding or purging, or the risks of gruesome surgery and subsequent infection, it was easier to take a few swigs of a proprietary medicine that promised to cure almost every ailment. If the patient did not have some serious or life-threatening disease, these remedies may indeed have been safer than some of the other contemporary conventional treatments. To many people, dosing one's self or family with a patent medicine that promised a guaranteed cure for almost everything seemed more reasonable than undergoing one of the less attractive conventional treatments that were available.

Medicine Shows

The traveling medicine show consisted of entertainment and sales pitches that were presented for the purpose of selling a particular brand of patent medicine. The American medicine show had its origins in the Middle Ages in Europe with traveling troupes of entertainers that sold patent medicines.

Medicine shows to sell proprietary nostrums were patterned after the older traveling shows that paraded acrobats, clowns, minstrels, and musicians around the country, stopping in small towns to amuse anyone who would attend. In many small towns, traveling medicine shows were a primary form of entertainment. People often came from miles around to enjoy the show and see patent medicines being touted in a carnival-like atmosphere. And indeed this type of sales technique continued on and was used by the promoters of other types of unorthodox medicine. Two examples that will be mentioned later were the touring "lectures" given by doctors promoting phrenology, and the educational shows that demonstrated the alleged power of static electricity as a healing force.

The atmosphere of the patent medicine shows was a combination of circus, minstrel show, Wild West spectacular, and vaudeville. Any novelty act that might possibly draw an audience to hear the pitch from the salesman was used. Shows featured such diverse performers as sword-swallowers, fire-eaters, singing groups, acrobats, snake-charmers, minstrels, musicians with lively tunes, and comedians with jokes. Attendance was free, but at various times throughout the show the entertainment was intermingled with commercial breaks for a salesman to present a sales pitch for the products with a rapid patter that was a combination of entertainment and sales. Medicine shows traveled from town to town in wagons, and later by train, from about 1850 until the 1930s.

Several factors helped to create the boom in the patent medicine business. Expansion of the railroad system into small towns across the country brought more salesmen and medicine shows, expansion of the postal system made ordering easier and sped delivery of the medicine directly to the home, and a sharp increase in the number of newspapers in small towns across the country in the late 1800s produced advertising to constantly persuade the consumer to buy the product.

The use of a patent medicine often gave the outward appearance of curing a particular disease or diseases. Most of them contained a high percentage of alcohol, and some contained opium or cocaine, thus the user might enter into a drug-induced haze and would indeed temporarily feel better.

The danger for the consumer was that someone would swig a patent medicine instead of going to a regular doctor and use of the quack elixir would interfere with the appropriate proper medical treatment. Some patients might feel better and continue to self-dose themselves, even though they continued to have the original disease. Thus the disease would progressively become worse, while the patient could well have been treated and cured by conventional medicine. An example of this was the use of Dr. King's New Discovery for Consumption, which claimed to be "the only sure cure for consumption in the world." The primary ingredients were morphine and chloroform. The chloroform stopped the coughing of the tuberculosis and the morphine put the user into a complacent frame of mind. In the meantime, the tuberculosis continued to ravage the lungs, but the victim felt no need for further treatment as he or she was not coughing and felt relatively good.

The same was true of quack medical devices. The user might think they were being effectively treated while they were actually receiving ineffective therapy, or no treatment at all, and possibly becoming worse.

Quack Doctors

Humbug, charlatan, con artist, swindler, and trickster. The quack doctor was someone who offered medical advice and treatments that were not necessarily based on medical or scientific knowledge or principles. Damian Thompson has claimed that the quack doctors of Georgian England were shameless liars and self-publicists. Often they awarded themselves phony degrees and other professional qualifications from institutes that existed only in their own imaginations.[6]

The pitchman, or pitch doctor, was the one who ran the medicine show and performed the sales spiel or "pitch." To add credibility to the sales pitch, the pitchman maintained an impressive appearance. Pitch doctors were typically distinguished-looking older men with a scholarly appearance, often with white hair and a smooth, professional way of conducting themselves. They dressed in a professional-looking

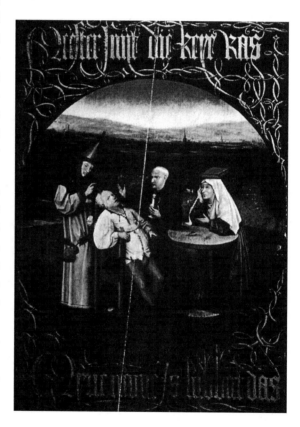

This scene of a quack doctor at work at his stand in a town on market day illustrates a treatment for insanity. A common belief in medieval times was that the removal of a "stone" from the head of a sick person would cure someone who was suffering from idiosyncrasies such as madness, folly, or deceit. The "doctor" is using a primitive scalpel to probe a surgical wound on the top of a seated man's head while two observers look on with curiosity (National Library of Medicine).

manner in a black Prince Albert frock coat and a silk top hat, in the manner of the physicians of the day, in order to look the part of an important "doctor." This imposing appearance was part of the act to sell to naïve and gullible audiences, which was exactly what they wanted to achieve. Many of the salesmen awarded themselves bogus medical degrees and called themselves "Doctor" or "Doc" to try to add some credentials for recommending and selling the product.

The quack himself usually had a charming and reassuring personality, and could produce user testimonials and explanations couched in pseudo-science to back up the product. The members of the medicine show entertainment troupe doubled as salespeople between acts and sold as much as they could by moving among the gathered crowd and showing the wares. Shills, confederates of the pitchman, might start the sales rolling by eagerly buying the first bottles of elixir or boxes of pills when the pitchmen held them up. Other shills in the crowd might yell out that they had been "cured" of some dread disease by this particular remedy.

The medical device quacks mostly fell into one of two general groups. The first were the charlatans who were deliberate con artists who knew that their cures didn't work. They would often lie about their credentials and make up success stories and glowing testimonials. The second group were those who had a poor understanding of scientific principles, but sincerely believed that their remedies worked. Both groups would exaggerate or mislead their patients, and often claimed that their remedies worked miracles in spite of the inability of contemporary science to provide the mechanism of action. These "cures" were ineffective at best, and deadly at the worst.

Quack Medical Devices

Dubious medical care was not restricted to patent medicines. The discovery and legitimate uses of magnetism, electricity, and radioactivity were quickly followed by their incorporation into a host of medical devices, many of which had no legitimate scientific or medical basis. Part of this was due to the aura surrounding new discoveries and their use in medicine, and partly because these devices appeared to "do" something, in the case of electrical devices usually by creating a mild burning or tingling sensation in the skin.

The inability of contemporary medicine to cure many diseases, such as typhoid, typhus, malaria, diphtheria, and measles, led people to try almost anything, legitimate or otherwise. Patients chose between regular medical treatment and treatment with a patent medicine or fringe medical device based on the seriousness of their illness, their proximity to a doctor, the cost of treatment, and how closely the sales pitch mirrored what the individual wanted to hear.

A medical device or treatment was quackery if it didn't conform to well-established laws of science or medicine, and the explanation for its action was based on principles that didn't hold up under scientific examination. In many instances, as we shall see, many devices and machines were based on questionable scientific principles that did not exist or certainly could not be proven in controlled laboratory studies by qualified scientific researchers. Another tip-off was when the described method of action of the treatment machine used fancy meaningless pseudo-scientific jargon that did not have any rational scientific basis, such as the example for the German patent medicine from the 1600s quoted above.

Marketing for bogus medical devices was important. Quackery was a type of medicine that was promoted through the spoken and the printed word. The smooth talk of a salesman, reinforced by reassuring advertising, sold many of these devices. The cost of going to a doctor and the uncertainty of a cure led many to seek self-treatment, buying devices at a local pharmacy or through mail order. Particularly popular were products that related to improving the user's sexual appeal or which offered the promise of attracting the opposite sex.

People purchased quack medical devices for many of the same reasons that they consulted licensed physicians; however, they also purchased them because the individual was embarrassed by the condition that needed treating. Common reasons were to lose weight, to cure baldness, or to improve outward appearance. Very often the reasons were to seek relief from chronic conditions for which conventional physicians had not provided a cure, such as persistent headaches or back pain, to relieve anxiety or depression, to increase overall strength or vitality, or to enhance sexual ability and raise the level of passion. Some unfortunates, on the other hand, were seeking cures for life-threatening illnesses. The quacks were always sympathetic and optimistic, claiming almost miraculous powers that achieved unfounded spectacular cures and resulted in stupendous success rates.[7]

Quacks often used or sold highly scientific-looking machines that appeared impressive from the outside. Many devices used colored indicator lights, made impressive mechanical noises, and contained numerous knobs, switches, and dials that may or may not have been connected to anything inside the machine or that had any functional action. It should have been fairly obvious that a machine should be suspect if the equipment didn't appear to do anything either mechanically or medically. Some of the more impressive machines produced mild electric shocks to the skin or vibrated the patient's body, as these actions appeared to the user to be positive evidence that the device was "doing something."

Bob McCoy, the founder and original curator of the Museum of Questionable Medical Devices in Minneapolis, concisely summed up several characteristics of a quack medical device. It was a machine that used a little-known form of energy that could not be detected by conventional scientists. The machine was capable of curing or diagnosing illness remotely or from a distance. The machine had a convoluted, impressive, "scientific-sounding" name. It was invented by a "world-famous" doctor that nobody had ever heard of. The manufacturer wasn't exactly sure how the device worked and was unwilling to explain its method of action. The machine had lights, knobs, and dials that didn't do anything. The machine shook, shocked, or warmed the body. The patient had to face a certain direction or use the machine at unusual times of the day. The machine was represented to cure anything. Customers were supposed to use the machine routinely for general health maintenance. The device was only available through the mail from the factory or through the company's agents. Finally, the device was not used or recommended by conventional doctors.[8] As described in later chapters, a great many bogus medical devices met one or more of these criteria.

Some quacks relied on what appeared at first glance to be "common sense" explanations to persuade customers that the machine was effective. Some compared themselves to renowned scientists. Others used "scientific-sounding" descriptions or complicated terms that sounded scientific to the general layman. To back this up, most manufacturers could provide impressive testimonials for how well the device worked and personal stories from people who claimed to have been cured. The origin and authenticity of these testimonials was often questionable.

Some companies augmented sales efforts with aggressive salesmen who traveled town-to-town selling their devices. Other common factors of quackery were that the manufacturer or salesman promised quick, easy, and painless results through the use of his device, scientific evidence that contradicted claims made for the device was ignored, scientific evidence that supported the sales claims was lacking, the sources of glowing testimonials were questionable, the device was sold door-to-door by aggressive salesmen or through the mail, and this was a revolutionary new machine that was allegedly more advanced than any of those known to conventional medicine. As part of the sales pitch, a common complaint to the consumer was that other doctors and scientists were not accepting the innovative technology of the device or taking the inventor's work seriously.[9]

Two of the Odder Ones

Two medical devices deserve special mention at this point, because they were indeed two of the odder devices that were successfully sold to an unsuspecting and gullible public, and they were both obvious frauds.

The Solarama Electron Therapy bed board, sold by a company in Greenville, South Carolina, consisted of paneling that contained metallic particles between sheets of asbestos. The board was intended to be placed between the mattress and box springs on a bed, so that it could treat the consumer while he slept. According to the manufacturer, the design was "based upon the principle of free electrons."[10] Whatever that was. Claims were that the board would treat fatigue, tension, backache, tiredness, headaches, ulcers, and benefit emotional tone. Even more optimistic were the claims for treating hemorrhoids, kidney infections, and high blood pressure. On January 7, 1975, the Food and Drug Administration ruled that the labeling provided "inadequate direction for such uses since worthless for such uses."[11]

The other example was an unusual device for assisting hearing that sold for $2, and was made by the Help-to-Hear Company of New York. The device consisted of a small piece of hard rubber that was placed against the teeth, with a wider side pointed towards the source of sound that the user wanted to hear. Needless to say, investigation showed that the device was useless for improving the hearing. The Help-to-Hear "Company" consisted of a young woman who mailed out sales literature from a rented desk at the address given in their advertising. Fraud orders against the company were issued in 1906.[12]

Quack or Questionable?

Legitimate physicians were supposed to have a legitimate university degree in medicine. Many quacks, however, called themselves "Doctor," even though they didn't have any formal degree. In some cases their medical degree came from a diploma mill or from a "medical school" that specialized in churning out students, mostly for a fee. Thus the quacks and charlatans promoting these devices often possessed no medical abilities, medical degrees, or diplomas, and often were not even licensed to practice medicine.

There were, however, exceptions to these generalities. Some of the promoters of questionable medical devices and practices were well-respected physicians, scientists, and educators. As the field of medicine was largely unscientific as the 1800s progressed, legitimate physicians often promoted ideas that, viewed from today's medical perspective and today's scientific light, were worthless if not even harmful. Until bacteria and viruses were proven to be the cause of most common diseases, physicians could only experiment and use trial-and-error methods to try to cure their patients.

Surprisingly, John Harvey Kellogg, a renowned surgeon and medical director of the world-famous Battle Creek Sanitarium, and Vincent Preissnitz, the founder of the successful water cure system, are now considered by some authors to be quacks.[13] This categorization, however, is somewhat unfair as they were both applying the latest medical knowledge of the day to try to benefit their patients. And indeed they were successful in treating many cases. The treatments administered by

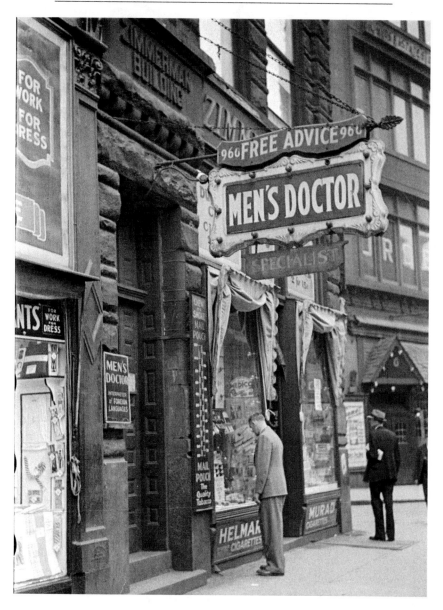

This photograph, taken by Arthur Rothstein in 1938, labeled "Quack Doctor, Pittsburgh, Pennsylvania," shows the exterior of an establishment that bears the hallmark of unconventional treatments with the signs that say "Men's Doctor" and "Free Advice." Shady practitioners offering private treatments for impotence and other "men's secret diseases" were consulted by hopeful individuals who did not want to undergo the embarrassment of consulting the family doctor (Library of Congress).

Preissnitz and at the Battle Creek Sanitarium and other Victorian spas were generally not harmful and, even though many were not perhaps particularly effective, most patients felt better for their treatments.

Though most quacks adopted a somewhat casual approach to the truth, they ranged from true believers in their products to fraudulent promoters of obviously bogus devices. But, in addition, medical devices and therapies that are considered today to be questionable or bogus were not always based on deception, and not all peculiar devices were bogus. Some were considered to be the latest technology that their inventors truly believed worked and were promoted by reputable doctors. So perhaps a better definition of a quack medical therapy, as stated by Kang and Pedersen is, "The practice and promotion of intentionally fraudulent medical treatments."[14] This included treatments and therapies that were based on claims for which there was no medical or scientific evidence.

For these reasons, the distinction between a quack and a regular medical practitioner was sometimes unclear. As mentioned in Chapter One, there was little regulation on medical practitioners in the 1800s, and certainly none on quacks.

The Power of Advertising

The late 1800s and early 1900s saw a shift in the way that consumer medical devices were marketed, with many of these health products being sold direct to the consumer. This shift is sometimes referred to as the rise of the medical marketplace.

Advertising and sales of quack medical equipment encompassed many devices, including competing brands of magnetic corsets, electrical stimulators and "invigorators," devices to drive oxygen into the body, electrical belts, magnetic socks, electric shock machines, and a host of other devices. Some were highly personal, such as breast and penis enlargers and prostate treatment devices, the nature of which readily lent themselves to mail-order sales to avoid embarrassing visits to a family doctor or neighborhood pharmacy.

The patent medicine industry pioneered American advertising techniques and strategy, and the sellers of bogus medical devices quickly learned and applied the same techniques. Patent medicine producers were experts in advertising and developing innovative ways of appealing directly to the consumer with sales methods that used exaggeration, deception, and psychological manipulation. Patent medicines and quack medical devices competing for the consumer's dollars had to continually advertise to keep their products on the forefront of consumer consciousness. With a large growth in the number of newspapers in the nineteenth century, patent medicine advertising and the industry flourished. Bogus medical device sales quickly followed in its steps.

Device sales did not rely solely on newspapers and magazines. Manufacturers of both patent medicines and medical devices used every means of advertising possible. They distributed educational pamphlets and calendars, presented sales talks disguised as "educational lectures," and wrote books that focused on the use of their products. Some manufacturers wrote medical manuals intended for either home or professional use that were partly instructional and partly advertising for the product. Many of the promoters went on the lecture and entertainment circuit, presenting popularized shows that combined science and pseudo-science with magic-lantern slide presentations and entertaining sales talks. These medical shows and lectures mixed science with showmanship, nominally to educate the public, but primarily to sell products. Though this seems like quackery and harks back to the patent medicine shows, some presenters provided serious demonstrations of their products, such as the use of static electricity machines or phrenology devices.

Given the lack of trust in doctors and their questionable ability to cure disease in the late 1800s, manufacturers of patent medicines advertised their wares with clever marketing psychology. Unscrupulous manufacturers produced medicines and devices that they felt would cater to the craving of the uneducated masses to have a simple, cheap, effective cure that they could use themselves at home. Manufacturers created a product and then created a demand for it by intense advertising campaigns. Advertising was often aimed at wives and mothers, who were usually the ones who were in charge of medical and nursing care for the family.

A favorite medium of advertising was the penny newspapers that emerged in the 1830s to report sensational tabloid news. These were a perfect match, as some of the medical claims for suspect devices were just as sensational as the news stories that accompanied them. Advertising for bogus medical devices appealed to the common man and woman by exploiting every human need and emotion.

By the late 1800s advertising in newspapers, magazines, and mail-order catalogs heavily promoted quack medicines and medical devices, along with questionable medical advice. The claims and cures were limited only by the copywriters' imaginations.

A significant role in advertising was played by fear. Two important ones were a fear of incurable illness (until the advertisement explained that the "cure" was here and could be purchased for a modest price via mail order) and a fear of sexual rejection. Themes of death, disease, and suffering were widely exploited. Manufacturers deliberately invented vague nonsensical descriptions of peculiar-sounding imaginary ailments for use in their advertising, such as "catarrh of the liver," "turbid biliousness," "acid fermentation," and "atonic dyspepsia."

Respectable popular magazines of the time, such as *Harper's Magazine, Collier's*, and *Atlantic Monthly*, carried full-page advertisements for patent medicines and for questionable medical devices. Estimates are that by the 1870s one-fourth of all print advertising was for patent medicines. In 1900 an editorial from the American Medical Association claimed that fully one-third of the advertising space in one of the Chicago newspapers consisted of advertisements for quacks and quack medicine.[15]

Most were bold advertisements that contained false statements about the effectiveness of a treatment and questionable testimonials to support their supposed effectiveness. Testimonials from satisfied users who said that they had been cured made the treatment appear to be more successful than it actually was. Unfavorable testimonials were presumably not used. Surprisingly, however, Dr. Arthur Cramp of the American Medical Association, who investigated many bogus claims in the early 1900s, said that contrary to the belief that most testimonials were faked or paid for, he felt that most were genuine. He thought that most were made in good faith, though he said they were often edited before publication.[16]

Manufacturers spent hundreds of thousands of dollars in advertising to convince the public that they had to rush out and purchase their particular product or to immediately send away for it in the mail. Part of the psychology of the quack manufacturers was that most of the readers of their advertising liked to read vivid and morbid descriptions of illnesses. If the advertising copy was cleverly worded, many of the readers would agree that they probably had some of these same symptoms. So they purchased the cure.

Advertisements were placed in national and local papers, handed out on street corners, and delivered by door-to-door salesmen. Most entrepreneurs were more versed in self-promotion than the sciences, thus much of the advertising showed a lack of scientific knowledge and a tendency towards hyperbole. However, one indication of the effectiveness of such advertising is that by 1902 patent medicines comprised 20 to 25 percent of all the prescriptions written in New York.[17]

Another deceptive practice in advertisements was to feature the photograph of a large building in some big city that was supposedly the company headquarters. The photograph did indeed legitimately show a large building in a busy city; however, it was often retouched before printing and the name of the bogus company was added somewhere onto the photograph, such as over the front door of the building, in order to make it seem like the company was much larger and more impressive than it really was.

Many manufacturers of questionable medical devices advertised their products and sold them directly through the mail. A typical Sears, Roebuck catalog had twenty pages of medicines, trusses, and other products guaranteed to cure everything from the common cold to cancer.[18]

Federal Regulation

Regulation of medical devices, whether legitimate or otherwise, has always been difficult. Even though laws were enacted to protect the public and the consumer from fraudulent medical devices, enforcement was traditionally an uphill battle. Proof of fraud was difficult, and in many instances fraudulent promoters who felt that the law was catching up to them simply closed up their business and opened up somewhere else under a different name. In some fraud cases quacks continued to operate in defiance of court orders and, in some instances, the entire process of shutting them down literally took decades. Lack of staffing at federal agencies to pursue quacks was always a problem.

Three agencies had differing degrees of authority to control the flood of fraudulent medical devices that enticed consumers. First, the United States Post Office had the authority to take action against anyone using the mail to defraud customers. Because many questionable devices were sold through mail order, this was one way to shut down fraudulent companies; however, the process could take years. The second agency was the Federal Trade Commission (FTC), which had the authority to take action against false and misleading advertising; however, again, proving a case and taking effective legal action against a company could be a lengthy process. In addition, the product or advertising had to involve interstate commerce, so products only sold locally did not fall under their jurisdiction.

The third and most important agency was the U.S. Food and Drug Administration (FDA). The regulation of medical devices in the United States today lies primarily under the jurisdiction of the FDA, although this was not always the case. In the late 1800s there were no federal regulations in place to prevent fraudulent medicines or medical devices from being advertised, promoted, and sold. The flood of bogus medical promotion was boosted by advertising in the daily and weekly newspapers and magazines.

Advertisements created fear in consumers and a feeling that they were riddled with disease by describing in detail some ghastly ailment that could attack the average person, then they offered a simple and easy cure with a particular medicine or device.

When the Pure Food and Drug Act came into law in 1906, patent medicines were an industry worth $80 million a year. Most patent medicines cost around eight to ten cents a bottle to produce, but as they sold for a dollar or more, this was a very profitable industry and attracted a variety of people to the money to be made.

Before the passage of the Federal Food, Drug and Cosmetic Act of 1906 and the Harrison Narcotic Act of 1914, the manufacturers of patent medicines were essentially free to promote and sell whatever they wanted. The Federal Food, Drug and Cosmetic Act was passed in 1906 to regulate food and drugs to ensure that they were manufactured to appropriate standards of purity.

President Theodore Roosevelt signed the Federal Pure Food and Drug Act in June 1906, and it went into effect January 1, 1907. The Act was passed into law after the publication of journalist Upton Sinclair's novel *The Jungle* (1906), a scathing exposé of unsanitary conditions in the meat packing industry, even though creating legislation was not Sinclair's intent. His original intention was to describe the harsh living and working conditions for working-class immigrants. Only part of the book described the meat industry, but it was that part that caught the attention of the public.

For the first time, the Act required the accurate labeling of food and drugs, and prohibited the shipment of adulterated food and drugs in interstate commerce. The Act required that the labels of drugs containing dangerous ingredients such as narcotics, in the form of alcohol, cocaine, opium, and morphine, indicate the presence, amount, and strength of these substances. The Act impacted the patent medicine industry because it required patent medicine makers to list the ingredients on their product labels, and prohibited the false or misleading labeling of the ingredients of medicine.

The 1906 Act, however, did not prohibit false therapeutic claims. The Pure Food and Drug Act of 1906 only regulated false and misleading labels, unsafe ingredients in food, and the adulteration of medical and food products. Patent medicine manufacturer's labels could say whatever they wanted, but they had to be true. It was a case of "buyer beware." It was up to the public to read the label and then decide if they wanted to take the medicine.

The Harrison Narcotic Act, passed in 1914, regulated the manufacture, importation, sale, and use of opium, cocaine, and other narcotics. There were exceptions in the federal law for small amounts of these drugs, but some states overruled the exemptions and maintained tight restrictions on all narcotics. Unfortunately the law only extended to the label on the product. It did not apply to advertising material, which was initially in print form in newspapers, then later as the spoken word on the radio. And, of course, advertising was the primary method to persuade potential customers to buy the product, thus patent medicine and device manufacturers continued to exploit a trusting and poorly-informed public. Copywriters based many of their claims on bogus or pseudo-scientific "facts," or simply made them up. Advertising copy was written to be manipulative, persuasive, and deceiving, and usually contained eye-catching drawings or photographs, often of consumers allegedly before and after using the medicine.

The Federal Trade Commission (FTC) was established in 1914 to monitor and regulate exaggerated and misleading advertising; however, it was not particularly successful in stopping the flood of false claims.

In 1928 the federal government authorized the Food, Drug, and Insecticide Administration to work with the Pure Food and Drug Act. In 1930 the agency was changed to the Food and Drug Administration (FDA). The FDA had the power to inspect factories, and to scientifically test food and drugs.

The FDA's authority to control medical devices and cosmetics was extended with the Federal Food, Drug, and Cosmetic Act of 1938. The current section 201(h) of the Food, Drug, and Cosmetic Act defines a medical device as an "instrument, apparatus, implement, machine, contrivance, implant, in vitro reagent, or other similar or related article, including a component part, or accessory which is … intended for use in the diagnosis of disease or other conditions, or in the cure, mitigation, treatment, or prevention of disease, in man or other animals."[19]

The 1938 Food, Drug, and Cosmetic Act significantly increased the government's regulatory authority over drugs and stiffened the penalties for those who broke the law. The Act further mandated pre-market reviews of the safety of new products, and banned false therapeutic claims in drug labeling.

The Act gave the FDA more power to regulate labeling, but the regulation of advertising remained with the FTC. Thus the process of filing a complaint against a manufacturer for misleading advertising, then dealing with the response, conducting hearings, and filing a cease-and-desist order, could take months or even years.

The effects of this legislation have been that cosmetic and therapeutic devices are currently regulated by the FDA. Manufacturers must provide scientific proof that new products are safe to use before putting them on the market, companies cannot "misbrand" products with false or inaccurate labels, and the FDA has authority to inspect factories that produce medical products. Anything other than low risk medical devices, such as tongue depressors and bedpans, must be approved by the FDA, and the FDA has the authority to seize illegal (e.g., mislabeled) medical devices and bring charges against those involved.[20]

THREE

Promises and Placebos

The reasons why people wanted to be treated by promoters of peculiar therapies, and why they purchased their bogus medical devices, involved a complex interplay between science, pseudo-science, and quackery. Basically, people started to seek alternative treatments and cures because the conventional medicine of the time did not necessarily heal. One example of the new medicine was the Victorian spa, which became the latest fad and trend of the late 1800s and early 1900s. At the time, drugs such as penicillin and the antibiotics now used to fight bacterial infections had not yet been developed, so physicians had to use whatever means of treatment were available. The use of mineral water for drinking and bathing appeared to be beneficial for some chronic ailments and, as a result, water treatments came into popular use.

Many people who tried out the latest mail-order medical devices of the late 1800s were looking for a cure for chronic ailments, because they had not been satisfied with the lack of results using the treatments offered by conventional mainstream medicine. In many instances they were looking for a cure for a longstanding problem. Many ill people were so desperate to find a cure that they would try anything, but some simply preferred to treat themselves at home with more convenience and at a lower cost than going to a doctor. Most of the therapies offered cures at home without pain, surgery, or often even consulting a doctor, all of which was what many consumers desired. In addition, many manufacturers offered advice through the mail. In this way worried consumers could get free advice without going to a doctor, thus avoiding the cost of treatment and embarrassment over sensitive personal problems.

Newspaper and other advertising for many of these bogus therapies fed on universal fears and anxieties about body image, diet, lifestyle, and chronic illnesses by offering quick and easy healing therapies. For women, the fear was often a fear of aging and a loss of sex appeal, while for men it was often a fear of the inevitable loss of sexual potency with aging.

Science Versus Pseudo-Science

Many of the bogus medical devices sold by mail-order claimed to cure all sorts of ailments, often presenting only very flimsy evidence for a successful cure in the form of a sales pitch and glowing testimonials. One of the indicators of quack medicine was that the treatment relied on anecdotal evidence for a cure, backed by misinformation that was packaged to look like scientific fact.[1]

Pseudo-scientists flourished prominently in the field of medicine more than any other because consumers had trouble distinguishing medical pseudo-science from real science, particularly in such a highly technical field. Thus medical quacks who gave themselves impressive-sounding credentials and spouted a pseudo-scientific theory did very well. Even worse, if they were sincere and really believed in their own therapy and what they were doing, they amplified their own delusions and belief in their own ideas.

Many of the promoters of quack medical products were distinguished-looking and talked with great authority about their own theories and important work. Some had legitimate diplomas and many were legitimate doctors. Unfortunately for mainstream physicians and the general credibility of the entire field, some of these fringe practitioners had degrees from small or alternative medicine schools, such as eclectic or homeopathic colleges, some of which were no longer in existence. Others were institutes that had been founded by the promoters so that they could award degrees to themselves.[2]

Spontaneous Cures

It would seem only logical to assume that many promoters of quack products could not succeed, given the ineffectiveness of many of their medical devices that had no apparent curative ability. However, often they flourished and made their fortunes.

There were two secrets to the success of bizarre and even ineffective medical devices and therapies. One was that many human ailments are self-limiting and eventually cure themselves, given sufficient time. Physicians generally agree that perhaps as many as 80 percent of all human illnesses, even if left untreated, will cure themselves through the normal defense mechanisms of the body. Thus, no matter what therapy was applied, if not harmful, the condition would resolve itself anyway. Many of these self-limited diseases simply ran their course, supported by adequate nourishment, fluid intake, rest, and warmth. As medical historian James Whorton has aptly pointed out, "the common cold will last a week if no medication is taken but be cured in seven days if drugs are used."[3]

Even the treatments of Heroic Medicine appeared to be "doing something" and, due to the fact that many diseases were self-limiting, many patients recovered from their illnesses in spite of the brutal treatments. The implication of this is that any treatment, if it is not harmful, will probably allow the majority of ailing people to return to a healthy state, given enough time to heal.

If some positive-sounding treatment was administered, whether through drugs, medical devices, or reassuring words, this action probably helped to stimulate the healing response and the likelihood of recovery was improved. A 1967 study in the *British Medical Journal* reported that patients with distressing symptoms, but no observable organic pathology, recovered at a rate of 64 percent when a diagnosis was made and the physician assured them that they would feel better in a few days, versus 39 percent for no treatment being administered.[4]

The other important factor was that many physical symptoms of human ailments are temporary or cyclical, occurring naturally from time-to-time, then disappearing and perhaps recurring again later. If some patients treated with quack devices had one of these chronic conditions that come and go, treatment may have coincided with the remission of symptoms. Thus, if symptoms spontaneously subsided after a certain treatment, no matter how peculiar or ineffective it was, patients (and even doctors) often inaccurately concluded that the treatment was responsible for their cure. In the absence of therapies with scientifically-proven effectiveness, the exact therapy made little difference in this era of hit-or-miss cures.

The Power of the Placebo

Scientific medicine tends to work best on definite diseases that can be diagnosed and pinpointed, and not as well on illnesses that lack obvious physical causes, particularly those of psychological origin. Thus another factor that contributed to the success of quack treatments was the placebo effect, which may have played a part in the acceptance of

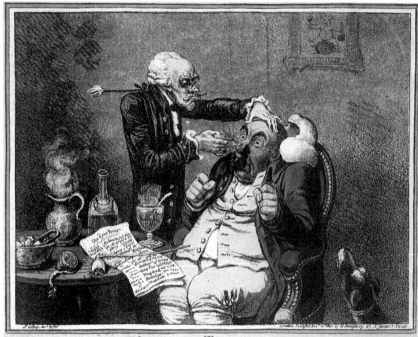

METALLIC-TRACTORS.

The power of the placebo should not be discounted. In 1795 Dr. Elisha Perkins of Connecticut claimed that he could cure internal diseases and speed the healing of wounds via the use of two metallic rods that he called "tractors." This painting titled "Metallic Tractors," made by James Gillray in 1801, shows Perkins "drawing" pain out of a patient with his metallic rods. Though now considered to be quack devices, they apparently helped some patients to cope with what may have been psychosomatic ailments (Wellcome Trust).

some of the odder therapies. The "placebo effect" occurs when a patient appears to improve, even though no treatment has taken place or an unconventional remedy that has no scientific or medical basis for success is used.

A placebo (from the Latin "I shall please") can be defined as an inactive substance or a procedure with no intrinsic therapeutic value, given or performed to satisfy the patient's psychological need for therapy. Studies of placebos have found that some people feel better and show measurable improvements after taking medicinal substances that have no demonstrable biochemical effect. Even the reassuring atmosphere of a doctor's office, the presence of a physician in a white coat, and some medical advice can produce a sense of relief and healing power in the patient. In many instances when a patient did not have a serious disease, the belief that something was being done to help them may have helped to effect a "cure."

The general public has routinely spent large amounts of money on questionable medical devices to treat everything from cancer to arthritis to baldness. Some of the devices that will be discussed in later chapters claimed to use special types of energy unknown to conventional science to effect a cure. Others rattled, shook, shocked, or vibrated the user towards better health. These various gadgets, with their special lights, heat, vibration, electric shocks, or radio waves, may have simply made the patient feel like the machine was doing something to cure them. Thus many medical procedures and treatments appeared to be effective, if believed by the patient to be "doing something."

The concept of relief of some illnesses gained with a placebo, particularly with ailments with a psychosomatic component, should not be taken lightly. Seemingly miraculous cures can occur simply due to a large amount of faith in a particular treatment or a particular doctor. In 1909 physician Samuel Gant commented, "Many Americans who suffer … are frequently cured while abroad because they have great faith in the ability of some celebrated physician of whom they have heard; consequently, at his suggestion they enter a hydrotherapeutic or other well-equipped institution, where they remain and take a systematic course of treatment with very beneficial results."[5]

The effect generated by placebos was recognized as far back as the sixteenth century. Most physicians believe and understand that the placebo effect is real, even if science cannot explain exactly how it works. Studies have confirmed the efficacy of placebos in almost every area of medicine.[6]

Placebo studies have found that some people can be helped or even "cured" merely by taking sugar pills. Author Cynthia Crossen has pointed out, "In almost all placebo-controlled studies, some of the placebo group will show improvements. In an August 1993 study of placebos, researchers found that two-thirds of patients receiving medically worthless treatments improved, even if temporarily."[7] Walter A. Brown, a psychiatrist at Brown University School of Medicine, wrote in 1998, "I believe that the placebo effect is a powerful part of healing and that more effort should be made to harness and enhance it."[8]

The placebo effect can be powerful and is generally accepted by modern medicine. About 30 percent of patients in clinical trials report feeling better after receiving a placebo.[9] Scientists are not sure how a placebo works, but the placebo effect is so strong that something is apparently triggered in the patient's brain that causes a physiological change. Possibly neurotransmitters are released that make the patient feel better. Gant commented that on many occasions he had administered colored water, bread pills, and other non-laxative agents to patients suffering from constipation, at the same time telling them that these were effective medicines. He said that in many cases the pills had the desired result the next morning. He also administered mild electric, mechanical, vibratory, and massage treatments to patients and "cured" them before they felt the application of the "treatment" had worn off.[10]

Sight, touch, and sound all tell a patient that treatment is being performed, even if they don't really understand what it is. Benefit may come from a compassionate caregiver, a sugar pill, or treatment by a complicated-looking machine.[11] Thus irregular therapies may have been useful in stimulating the placebo effect, even if that was not the intention.

The placebo effect has traditionally been an important tool for managing some conditions. For example, some of the therapies administered at Victorian-era sanitariums seemed to have a strong placebo effect, particularly for those with "nervous diseases" and psychosomatic illnesses. Even if science could not show any particular benefits from these treatments, the hands-on attention given by caring attendants may have had a powerful soothing and placebo effect. In many instances, people seeking curative spa treatments were helped simply by a change of scenery and a rest.

Gant, for example, felt that patients usually recovered faster when they stayed in a well-equipped sanitarium or hydriatic institute than when treated at home or in a physician's office.[12] He advised patients to soothe their nerves in pleasant surroundings and forget business worries. He felt that the power of suggestion often corrected nervous and other conditions that went along with their ailments. His point was that people receiving treatments for nervousness and other psychosomatic illnesses often had nothing physically wrong with them that could not be cured by attention and treatment from a caring health professional.

Practitioners who believe strongly in their treatments and administer them with confidence may do the patient some good through the powers of suggestion, reassurance, and imagination. Dr. Robert DeLap of the U.S. Food and Drug Administration has said, "Expectation is a powerful thing. The more you believe you're going to benefit from a treatment, the more likely it is that you will experience a benefit."[13]

Gant felt that it was important to listen to the patient and not belittle their symptoms. He told patients to keep regular hours, to abstain from excessive drinking, and spend a considerable amount of time in the open air, walking, playing golf, horseback riding, and exercising. He said that patients often created in themselves an exaggerated belief in the curative power of electricity, massage, and vibration treatments, and it apparently worked for them.[14]

Many people went to irregular practitioners for treatment of anxiety, chronic pain, and back problems. The placebo effect may have played a role in these instances. Some psychosomatic symptoms may have been alleviated merely because patients believed they would improve after undergoing treatments with complex machines. The humming, buzzing, electrical sparks, and mild shocks of some of the electrical machines used in the late 1800s and early 1900s may have been perceived by the patient as beneficial. In addition, using any type of treatment may have lessened the patients' fears and made them feel better emotionally, even if the physical symptoms persisted.

Proof of Effectiveness

The important question to ask when considering the use of a medical device to treat any human ailment is, does the device effect a cure? As discussed above, a "cure" may also occur due to spontaneous remission from the ailment or the condition may be improved by the placebo effect. How then do we know that the device or machine has improved the condition?

Two common errors occurred with the early alternative medical systems. One was the error that if a practitioner treated an ill patient and the patient recovered, the practitioner convinced himself that the treatment resolved the ailment. In other words the cure might be coincidental, but it was perceived as being causal. Faulty *post hoc, ergo propter hoc* reasoning argued that if patient improved after a certain treatment, then the treatment produced the cure.

One example of this was the origin of Thomsonian medicine, promoted by Samuel Thomson from New Hampshire in the late 1700s. After he persuaded a local farmer to eat some of the *Lobelia inflata* plant, the man vomited but claimed that his health had improved. Thomson used this "evidence" as a basis for his system of botanic cures. Unfortunately, Thomson fell into the common scientific trap of *post hoc* reasoning that if the patient recovered after taking his herbal medicine, the plant must have effected a cure.

The second major error made by fringe medical practitioners was to take a limited success and expand it to meet all situations. Treatment was based on the idea that if it helped some people under some circumstances, it could treat everything and cure everyone. This type of error was committed by Daniel Palmer, the originator of chiropractic. He manipulated the spine of a deaf individual and achieved an apparent cure for the man. He then advanced the theory that manipulation of the spine could cure many other ailments.

Clinical Trials

When investigating any form of treatment, a researcher is typically looking for cause-and-effect. In other words, does this particular treatment result in healing? Quacks rarely performed clinical trials as a scientist would, but preferred to rely on their own intuition and testimonials from satisfied users of their products. One of their biggest fallacies was the previously-mentioned *post hoc* reasoning.

Manufacturers of modern medical devices perform clinical trials in an attempt to determine whether treatment provided by a device or procedure produces a significant effect on the outcome for the patient. The basic question is, does using this machine or treatment help to relieve the condition it is intended to treat?

To determine the answer to this fundamental question, a researcher will assemble a group of suitable test subjects. Next, the subjects are typically divided into two groups, an experimental or treatment group and a control or non-treatment group. It is important that none of the subjects know which treatment they are getting and the participants do not know what results the experiment is hoping to find. Testing will therefore be set up as what is called a "blind experiment," in which the subjects participating in the testing are not aware whether they are part of the treatment group or the control group in order to remove any bias on the part of the subjects being tested.

The treatment group receives the experimental treatment. The other receives a placebo treatment that does nothing and is harmless. Both groups, however, appear to receive exactly the same treatment. For example, one group receives the medicine or therapy being tested while the other is given a placebo that appears to be just the same. At the end of the testing, the responses of the treatment group are compared to those of the control group to see if any difference is statistically significant, which simply means that the results are unlikely to have occurred merely due to chance.

A placebo is given to the control group to account for the placebo effect, by which patients receiving the placebo treatment may still report a positive effect as if they had been receiving the real treatment. The placebo effect may affect both the treatment and the control group. In the case of a drug trial, the treatment group would receive the drug, but the placebo group would be given a sugar pill. In the case of testing an electrical device for some form of shock treatment, the treatment group would receive the electrical shock, while the control group would undergo the same test procedure as the treatment group, but would not receive the shock.

Another problem in this type of research is that there can be possible bias on the part of the tester. If the researcher knows which subject belongs to which test group there can be possible bias in the test results, as the researcher may unconsciously be looking harder at the treatment group for positive results. This is resolved by what is called a "double-blind experiment," where subjects are assigned randomly to the control and experimental groups. Neither the researcher nor the subject know which group any of the subjects belong to until after the results are gathered.[15] One of the researchers on the project who is not involved in the testing knows, but will not identify which group each subject is in until the all the results are gathered. This safely removes any bias from both the primary researcher and the subjects.[16] A good experimental design uses a highly controlled environment to try and figure out which factor causes a change in the studied result and includes controls for variables that might adversely affect the results.

The number of people used in a particular study will affect the results. It is important to have a large enough number of subjects in the test and control groups to achieve accurate test results, to be able to feel confident in the results, and to be able to extrapolate the results to the entire population. The larger the number of test subjects, obviously the closer the group is to representing the entire population, in order to be able to generalize the conclusions. If the number of test subjects is too small, it is not possible to draw wide enough conclusions; however, too large a study group can also adversely affect the results. Statistical methods are used to determine the appropriate number of test subjects required to produce statistically-significant results.[17] To use the example of D.D. Palmer again, he drew his conclusions from a sample size of one, e.g., only one subject. This is not a large enough number to draw any significant conclusions. In statistical terms, "significance" means that the results that occurred were not due to random chance.

Finally, after the experiment is completed, it is necessary to apply proper data and statistical analysis in order to be able to draw the appropriate conclusions and to assure that the correct conclusions are being drawn. Some of the problems that can occur are that the results may be overstated, the conclusions aren't backed up by proper statistical analysis, or that the conclusions go beyond the discovered results and are mistakenly extrapolated to other test populations and different conditions.[18] The very mention of statistics makes most non-mathematicians cringe, but statistical analysis is a precise way to determine whether or not an experimental treatment is effective.

One of the hallmarks of quackery is that the claimed results cannot be duplicated and independently confirmed. Thus, another factor that is important for any clinical trials of a drug or medical device is that the results have to be repeatable by independent researchers.

This all sounds fairly simple and obvious, but it is much more complicated in practice. The experiment has to be designed well and valid comparisons made. It takes a series of repeated studies to replicate and confirm a hypothesis. If the studies do not support the hypothesis, then the hypothesis is wrong.

Here is a simple example of a potential error. Doctors observe that people who take vitamin C every day have fewer colds than those who don't take it. Is the conclusion that vitamin C prevents colds? Not necessarily. This conclusion is only an observation, not a scientific experiment. Perhaps the people who take vitamin C would have been just as healthy if they had not taken vitamin C. Perhaps these people eat healthier food, or they may exercise more and be generally healthier, they may stay away from crowds that are the source of colds, or they may wash their hands more often. A carefully designed experiment would have to be run to account for all these other variables. In an observational experiment, such as this one, there is no control over any of the other variables. This method might be good for a simple survey, but not for showing cause-and-effect relationships.[19]

In the example described above, there is nothing to use for comparison to the observed results. The correct method would be to perform a randomized double-blind test using a placebo for comparison, in which neither the researcher nor the subject know which treatment is which. If the vitamin C is more effective than the placebo, the results are evaluated with statistics. If the new treatment works no better than the placebo, then the proposed treatment essentially doesn't work.

The placebo effect helps to explain the apparent effectiveness of some cures, even if there are no reliable medical benefits. If more people regain health using a drug than those using a placebo, the drug is probably effective, but this requires complex statistical analysis to confirm the result.

Professional statisticians look at the data from an experiment and try to come up with a reasonable explanation for why the result occurred. Quacks sometimes used statistics to support their opinions. Unscrupulous quacks forced the data to fit their theories. They ignored other or contradictory facts, or even made up data to support their views.

Correlation measures the degree of relationship between two variables. The variables have a strong positive relationship if a high score on one variable is associated with a high score on the other variable.[20] But just because two variables are correlated and appear to be related to each other does not mean that one variable caused the other. As another example, studies have showed that there is a relationship between listening to classical music and intelligence. However, a researcher cannot say that listening to classical music causes higher intelligence. This is not a causal relationship. It may be just as likely that people who listen to classical music are more intelligent to begin with than to infer that the music has caused the increased intelligence.

Causation and correlation was one source of error that was common among quacks. A correlation study is when two variables are measured together in some setting. There is no random assignment of subjects to groups. If the two variables appeared to be related, many quacks assumed that one variable caused the other. The mistake is made when people infer causation from a correlation study.

Here is one example taken to the extreme. Everybody who dies has drunk water, thus the inference is that drinking water causes people to die. Therefore the erroneous conclusion drawn is, do not drink water. In a similar train of thought, many criminals drink alcohol, therefore the use of alcohol causes crime. These are absurdly simplistic cases, but it is easy to extrapolate the thinking to a medical case. For example, 50 percent of the people who received a type of electric shock treatment had their symptoms relieved, therefore giving shocks to people will relieve their symptoms. Of course some of the other factors to be considered are, what was their type of illness, how long had they had it, were they spontaneously cured, was it a placebo effect, and did they suffer any relapse?

A final factor to be considered when looking at the results of studies is to determine who paid for the study and what was their financial interest? Ideally, there should be no financial ties between the investigators and their studies. Obviously someone promoting their own product, such as a manufacturer of a quack device, will look to find the best possible results and they may even report only the positive results that they want to promote.

To sum up, when testing a new device or treatment procedure, it is essential to collect a sufficient number of clinical observations and to achieve a careful analysis of the results on a statistically valid number of patients in order for the results to be credible to the medical community. And this is something the promoters of quack medical devices didn't do.

Four

Some Early Medical Devices

Though most of the medical peculiarities described in this book were a product of the late 1800s and early 1900s when mechanical and electrical technology became more and more a part of contemporary life, legitimate devices used for medical purposes have been available for healers to treat human ailments since before recorded history. Roman surgical instruments used during medical treatment, such as knives and specula, have been found to date back to at least 79 AD.[1]

The stethoscope, a major medical device and diagnostic advance, was invented in 1816 by French physician René Théophile Hyacinthe Laënnec. To use this device, the physician placed one end of a rigid tube to his ear and the other to the patient's chest, and was thus able to hear heartbeats clearly. The tubes used on stethoscopes in poorhouses were often very long, so that the physician could keep his distance from any patients who might also be a carrier of fleas. The binaural version of the stethoscope with ear-pieces and flexible rubber tubing for use with both ears was not developed until 1852 by physician George Cammann.

Before the development in 1867 by Thomas Clifford Allbutt in England of a practical portable clinical thermometer similar to the modern clinical thermometer, a physician could only obtain a crude indication of a patient's body temperature and suspected fever by touching the patient's skin and using remembered experience. By 1880, physicians were starting to routinely use medical instrumentation for tasks such as pulse and temperature measurement in order to provide a more-precise and clearer understanding and diagnosis of diseases. However, even modern devices for measuring blood pressure were not perfected until the 1920s.[2]

Though most of this book concentrates on the bogus medical

devices that appeared in the late Victorian age, it is interesting to also look at a few of the earlier unusual devices used to treat human illness.

Amulets and Talismans

One of the first medical "devices" used for disease prevention and healing purposes was the amulet. The practice of carrying amulets or charms to bring good luck and good health through protection against disease has a long history. An amulet was a type of charm, often worn as a necklace, that had supposed magical powers and was used to protect against injury or evil, including disease and illness. Many amulets were phallic in shape, intended to induce fertility in the user.[3]

Ancient amulets were typically made from bronze or another metal, gemstones, ceramic, or similar materials that were believed to have magical powers to ward off illness or to effect a cure. For example, copper charms were carried in ancient Greece as protective amulets against smallpox in the 600s BC. Bone amulets in the form of a hand and arm, displaying a fig or *mano fica* gesture with the thumb between the index and second finger, were worn in Rome as late as the late 1800s to protect against the evil eye. A horse's tooth, worn on a necklace, was used in Algeria to cure pain and diseases of the breasts. A rabbit's foot, worn similarly, might be used for protection against rheumatism. In the southwestern United States, Native American medicine men used sacred turquoise amulets in diagnostic and healing rituals, and incorporated the ground-up gemstone into love potions.[4]

A talisman intended to prevent illness was supposed to have magical powers against evil, and was often made in the form of a ring or stone bearing engraved figures or important symbols, such as the beetle. Some Egyptian and Greek amulets were charms that were inscribed with magical texts and invocations for a particular cure. By carrying the healing ceremony itself in this form, the words did not have to be constantly repeated for the chronically ill, as the magical formula was continuously in contact with the wearer.

Not all use of amulets was for primitive medicine. In the late 1680s English physician William Read promoted a device named the Anodyne Necklace, which was a charm intended to help infants who were teething. Among his promotional material, Read claimed that Queen Anne used his wonderful necklaces for the royal children.[5] Others quickly jumped on the bandwagon. A promoter inappropriately named Maj. Choke also sold necklaces to help children who were teething. Anodyne necklaces supposedly made from the bones of St. Hugh additionally capitalized on the religious healing power of rosary-style beads and the bones of the saints.[6]

As the use of electricity became popular in medicine in the late 1800s, it was incorporated into teething cures, such as in Butler's Electro-Medical Teething Necklace.[7] This device appears in druggist's supply catalogs in 1922, but was banned as ineffective by the Post Office in 1947.

Madstones

Similar in intent to the use of amulets, a madstone, also called a bezoar, was a hard nugget of material that was thought to have magical powers. The bezoar was thought to be a remedy for snakebites, insect stings, and bites from rabid animals. For use, it was placed on the wound to "draw out" the poison.

A bezoar was not an actual stone or rock, but was a concretion found in the stomach or intestines of some mammals. It was a solidified mass that formed around a foreign substance in the animal's gastrointestinal tract, and was composed of an amalgamation of hair, mineral and vegetable matter, and other foreign material. In ancient Arabic medicine, the general category of bezoars included previously-expelled human gallstones and kidney stones.

Contracting rabies was inevitably fatal before the development of a suitable rabies vaccine developed by Louis Pasteur and Émile Roux in 1885. Prior to that time, a bezoar was a popular folk-remedy for the prevention and treatment of the disease. Part of the basis for using it as a cure was that rabies did not always develop after a bite from a rabid animal. Only approximately 30 percent of those bitten actually developed the disease. Death from rabies if contracted, however, was inevitable and was a horrible end, involving frothing at the mouth, violent movements, aggression, and agitation. Because of the frightening symptoms and the danger of contracting the disease, nobody wanted to care for rabies victims. Most of the victims who developed the disease were either locked in jail or otherwise kept in isolation until they died. Thus those who had been bitten by a rabid animal and potentially had the disease were willing to try anything, including the use of a bezoar.

This again was an example of faulty causal reasoning. The thinking was that because 70 percent of the people who were bitten used the bezoar and did not die, the bezoar must have been effecting a cure for the majority of the cases. The real reason, of course, is that the 70 percent who recovered did not develop the disease to begin with.

In the Middle Ages, bezoars were kept as a family heirloom and were passed down from generation to generation. Some might have been in the same family for as long as 150 years.[8]

Perpetual Pills

Another curious medical "device" that was treated as a family heirloom was the "perpetual pill" or "everlasting pill." In France in the 1770s, and well into the 1800s, pharmacists sold a small spherical pill to produce purging and vomiting that was made from metallic antimony, a poisonous heavy metal that was commonly used in Heroic Medicine. When the pill was swallowed, it produced an irritating purgative action. It passed unchanged through the digestive tract, and was later recovered, washed, and used again and again, thus earning their name. Perpetual pills were treated as family heirlooms and were often passed down from one generation to the next.

The Stone Doctors

In the Middle Ages mental illness was not understood and treatment of those with mental conditions was nonexistent or primitive. Mental illness was regarded as God's punishment for some evil deed that the person had committed, and the insane, like rabies victims, were typically hidden away out of the sight of mainstream society. Those with mental disorders were locked in prisons alongside criminals, in almshouses, or confined to the attic at home. Some people considered the insane to be possessed by evil spirits, and had demons that were often exorcised by violent means. One treatment for insanity was to apply a blistering agent to the shaven head of a mentally ill person to "draw out" the evil. Trephining, or drilling a hole in the skull to supposedly release the disease-causing demon, was also used.

A common belief in medieval times was that the removal of a "stone" from the head of a sick person would cure someone who suffered from traits such as madness, folly, or deceit. One well-known painting depicting this was created around 1494 by Dutch artist Hieronymus Bosch. The scene was called "Cutting the Stone," also known as "The Extraction of the Stone of Madness" or "The Cure of Folly." Bosch showed a doctor using a primitive scalpel to probe a surgical wound on the top of a seated man's head. In the painting Bosch changed the object being extracted from a stone to the bulb of a flower, possibly to hint that the doctor was a quack.

Plague Masks

Another early curious medical invention was the protective outfit used by plague doctors. Bubonic plague, the Black Death, haunted Europe until the beginning of the eighteenth century. Serious epidemics of the plague flared up in England every twenty years or so between 1347 and 1666. In 1665, more than 100,000 died in London alone. The plague reached a high point in Europe between 1347 and 1351 when it killed an estimated fifty million people.

The plague was spread by a bacillus carried by fleas on rats, which were prevalent in the filth of medieval cities and which jumped onto nearby likely victims to spread the disease. The Black Plague was highly contagious and virulent, and killed most of its victims within three days.

The popular children's nursery rhyme summed it up:

> *Ring-a-ring of rosies,*
> *A pocket full of posies,*
> *Atishoo, atishoo,*
> *We all fall down.*

Rosies were the purple patches that developed on the chest of the plague victim, *posies* referred to the nosegay of aromatic herbs and spices that were thought to protect from the plague, the sneezes were part of the symptoms, and the last line sums up what eventually happened to the victim because the disease did not have a cure.

Today medical personnel have isolation suits with self-contained air-filtering systems for use while treating highly-infectious patients. In the Middle Ages physicians without some form of protective measures were quite likely to contract communicable diseases from their patients. During the plague years doctors tried to protect themselves from contagion with birdlike headpieces and masks that featured beaks that projected up to eighteen inches in front of their faces. This gave them the sometime nickname of "beak doctors." These peculiar-looking outfits were first used by plague doctors in Paris during the early seventeenth century.

The long beak was intended to function as a crude

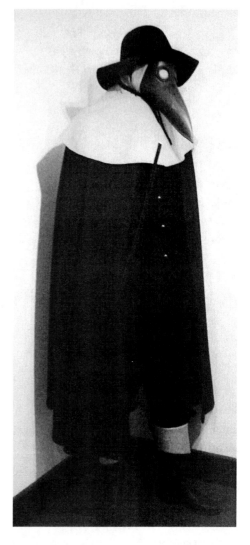

This was how medieval physicians dressed when treating the Black Plague. The long beak-like mask contained aromatic herbs that were thought to purify the air of disease so that the doctor could breathe safely. The black ankle-length overcoat was impregnated with wax or fat to seal out the plague germs. The long wooden "tickle stick" was to prod and poke the patient from a safe distance while trying to make a diagnosis (author's collection).

form of gas mask. Aromatic herbs and spices were stuffed into the beak to cleanse the "bad air" being breathed in. Eyeholes in the mask were often covered with glass that was tinted a red color in order to stare down the "evil eye" of the disease. To protect the rest of their bodies, plague doctors wore ankle-length overcoats that were smeared with wax or fat to seal the material from the disease, along with gloves, boots, and a tight-fitting hat.

Plague doctors typically carried a long wooden cane, nicknamed a "tickle stick," which allowed the doctor to prod and poke the patient from a safe distance while trying to make a diagnosis.[9]

One of the recommended remedies to guard against the plague was the use of amulets made from dried toads or lizards. Another supposed preventive was to fasten a bone taken from the head of a toad onto the chest of the victim.

Fleams and Scarificators

Bloodletting as a treatment technique had been used since before the time of the Greek physician Hippocrates to relieve supposed congestion within the body.[10] Primitive instruments used by early physicians to cut the skin to promote the escape of blood were animal bones, sharpened pieces of wood, or seashells with an edge ground to knife-like sharpness. In medieval Europe, blood-letting was performed by barbers and barber-surgeons because performing the procedure was considered to be below the dignity of physicians.[11]

The popular tool for bleeding that was used to open a vein in the eighteenth and nineteenth centuries was the lancet, a pointed steel surgical knife with two edges, about two-and-a-half inches long, mounted on the end of a wooden handle.[12] The device was also called a fleam. Some lancets were contained inside the handle and were spring-loaded, so that when a small lever or button on the side of the device was pressed, the blade sprang out and stabbed deep into the patient's flesh for better penetrating action. Some lancets folded like a pocketknife and some had three or more blades of different sizes. For obstinate cases, there was an accompanying wooden "fleam stick," which was used to hit the back side of the blade to drive it in further. The multi-bladed fleam was also used for bleeding horses.

The scarificator was another bleeding device. It consisted of a small brass box that contained anywhere from four to sixteen blades (typically ten or twelve) that acted at the same time to make multiple short cuts in the skin to draw out more blood. The device was spring-loaded in order to drive the blades firmly into the skin and make a series of shallow cuts. The scarificator was used until well into the twentieth century.[13]

Wet and Dry Cupping

Bleeding was sometimes accompanied by a procedure called "cupping" to promote the flow of blood. When used in combination with bleeding, this was called "wet" cupping.

Wet cupping used a series of five to seven glass cups that looked like whiskey shot glasses, of one to four ounce capacity (anywhere from the size of an eggcup to a small teacup). The cups had a special rim of thick glass to promote a good seal to the skin. After several incisions were made in the flesh with a lancet, the blood that collected at the surface was drawn out of the skin into the cups via a partial vacuum.[14]

Before use, the inside of the cup was heated with a candle or a spirit lamp, then applied to the skin in the desired location. As the glass cooled, it created a lowered air pressure inside the sealed cup and thus induced a partial vacuum that helped to accelerate bleeding and draw out the blood. Another method to create the vacuum was to rub the inside of the cup with alcohol. The alcohol was lit with a match to burn out the air in the cup and heat the glass. When the flames died away, the warm cup was placed on the skin over the cuts. As the glass cooled, the lowered pressure inside the cup created a partial vacuum and suction on the skin, and drew out the blood from the surface.

Another procedure called "dry" cupping used the same general technique without the incisions in the skin. In this technique the heated cups were applied in the same manner and left in place until the skin reddened as it promoted the flow of blood under the skin.

Medicinal Leeches

Though not strictly speaking a medical device, leeches were often used as part of the bleeding process to promote the removal of blood. The leech was a blood-sucking worm (*Hirudinea medicinalis*) found in wet earth, ponds, and farmlands. Leeches used for medicinal purposes preferably came from Sweden, as they had about six times the sucking power and capacity of American leeches.

For bleeding internal cavities, such as inside the mouth, a medical device called a leech tube was used. This was a tapered tube that was open at both ends. The leech was wedged in from the larger end, so that only its mouth protruded from the narrow end. This way the leech could not escape during treatments of the mouth and be swallowed during the procedure.[15]

Live leeches were stored before use in large decorative porcelain or glass jars. Leeches were sometimes temperamental after being stored and handled, and required some coaxing to get them going. Physicians often had to prick the skin to start them sucking. When the leeches were full, they dropped off naturally and were usually destroyed by covering them with salt and then burning them.[16] In earlier times, leeches were reused by economy-minded practitioners as long as they continued to suitably perform their task.

The Tobacco Smoke Resuscitator

In Europe in the 1600s and 1700s drowning, or near-drowning, was not an unusual occurrence, because swimming was not the popular pastime that it is today and the ability to swim was not universal. Many people drowned needlessly after falling into rivers, lakes, and canals, particularly in large cities, such as London, Paris, and Amsterdam, that were built around water.

Cardio-pulmonary resuscitation (CPR) was totally unknown at the time, and the only useful method for restoring circulation was to briskly rub of the body of a drowned person with hot cloths.

Artificial respiration was vaguely known. Samuel Auguste Tissot, a Swiss physician of the eighteenth century, recommended that the rescuer blow hard into the victim's mouth. At least one home medical manual from the mid-nineteenth century recommended an early method of mouth-to-mouth resuscitation when it described holding the victim's nose shut and blowing into the victim's mouth with as much force as possible to ventilate the lungs.[17]

Tissot believed, as did other eighteenth-century doctors, that the primary cause of drowning was not the inhalation of water, but the ensuing froth that it created inside the lungs. To counteract this, victims of near-drowning were treated with tobacco smoke via a pipe stuck into the mouth, as tobacco vapor was thought to dissolve this froth, thus allowing the lungs to resuscitate the victim naturally.

At the time, tobacco, the dried leaf of a series of plants in the *Nicotiana* family, was used as a medicine, primarily for the effects of the drug nicotine that tobacco contains. Nicotine in tobacco smoke had a strong stimulating effect, forcing the body to produce adrenaline, which was a heart and circulatory stimulant.[18] Nicotine was easily absorbed from the intestinal tract and liquid preparations of tobacco were routinely administered as an enema for a variety of conditions. In small doses the tobacco had a stimulating effect on the nervous system, particularly on the respiratory system. Thus medical reasoning was that a faster method to speed the introduction of tobacco smoke into the interior of a drowning victim was to force it into the rectum. Tobacco smoke applied in this manner was thought to warm the victim and stimulate the breathing.

The smoke was applied via a device named a "fumigator."[19] Tobacco leaves were burned in a small metal box that had a tube attached to each side of it. One tube ended in a nozzle that was inserted into the victim's rectum; the other was attached to a set of bellows that was used to blow the smoke into the patient. This technique was also used to revive lethargic new-born infants and women who had fainted, and to treat cases of asphyxiation.

Entire organizations were founded and dedicated to the study and practice of the resuscitation of drowned people. The first was the *Society for the Recovery of Drowned Persons*, founded in Amsterdam in 1767. Because of this, use of the tobacco smoke enema became known as "Dutch fumigation."[20] Dutch fumigation was considered to be such a valuable technique for the resuscitation of the drowned that it became the standard technique for treating victims of any water mishaps.

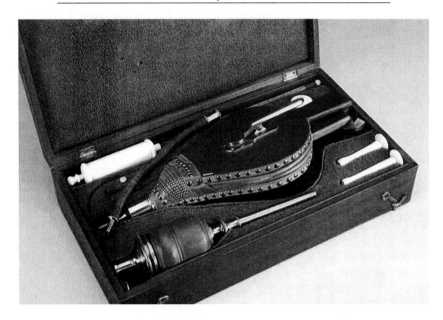

The medieval version of today's automated defibrillators, this set of resuscitation equipment, called a "fumigator," was designed to introduce tobacco smoke into individuals who were experiencing collapse from drowning. Tobacco was burned in the round device in the foreground and then injected with the bellows. The injected tobacco smoke was thought to produce a stimulating effect on the nervous and respiratory systems (The Science Museum, London, from the Wellcome Collection).

Special appliances with bellows for administering tobacco smoke were installed in public places near large bodies of water, such as coffee shops and barbershops on the banks of rivers, somewhat like the prevalence of AED (Automated External Defibrillator) devices today.

Similar organizations for resuscitating drowning victims were soon founded in Germany, Italy, Austria, France, and London. So many people drowned by falling into the River Thames in London that a society named *The Institution for Affording Immediate Relief to Persons Apparently Dead from Drowning* was formed in 1774 by Dr. William Hawes and Dr. Thomas Cogan to promote the resuscitation of drowning victims.[21] Later renamed the Royal Humane Society, the organization stationed equipment to carry out the procedure to revive the drowned along the waterfront in the 1880s, and trained residents of nearby houses on how to use it.

Today the development and widespread dissemination of the

techniques of CPR and automatic defibrillators have thankfully made this technique out of date, and the term "blowing smoke" remains today only as a vulgar expression for an insincere compliment.

Reviving drowning victims by treating their bowels was a common practice in the mid–1800s. If the fumigator failed, *The Ladies' Indispensable Assistant* recommended an enema of turpentine, a very irritating substance, to revive those who had nearly drowned.[22] Other stimulating treatments for drowning called for snuff or ginger to be blown up the nose.[23] Ancient Chinese medicine referred to blowing air into the ear with a tube to treat an unconscious patient.

Another technique for reviving victims of drowning, which must have been much easier and more discreet, was called the "hogshead" method. The victim was draped over the outside of a large barrel placed on its side, and the barrel was then rolled back and forth. The back-and-forth jostling motion was thought to force water to flow out of the drowned victim's lungs. Other physicians advised simply hanging the patient upside down to allow the water to flow back out.[24]

Metallic Pain Tractors

In 1795 Dr. Elisha Perkins of Connecticut announced to the Connecticut Medical Society that he could cure internal diseases and speed the healing of wounds via the use of two metallic rods and a system of medicine he called "tractoration." A highly regarded physician in New England, Perkins had noted that when his metallic instruments came into contact with muscles during surgery, the muscle contracted. He also noted that pain seemed to go away when metal instruments were used to separate the gums from the teeth during extractions.[25]

Perkins believed that illness was caused by too much electrical "fluid" in the afflicted parts. He reasoned that pain could therefore be relieved by discharging the excess undesired electrical energy with his metallic tractors. Legitimate scientific discussions of electromagnetism and induced currents that were prevalent at the time appeared to confirm his pseudo-scientific ideas. In 1796 Perkins applied for a patent for the Perkins Metallic Tractor for the relief of pain from headache, rheumatism, and other diseases. This was the first United States patent granted for a medical device.

Perkins' invention consisted of two rods made from different metals. Allegedly one rod was an alloy of copper, zinc, and gold, and the other was made from iron, silver, and platinum.[26] In reality, one was made from iron and the other from brass.[27] Both rods were about three inches long, tapering to a point at one end, and rounded on the other. Each tractor had a round profile on one side and was flat on the other, the entire device looking somewhat like the shape of a bisected carrot.

Perkins found that the same effect could be achieved with any metallic device, such as a penknife or metal comb, but he did not want people to use items commonly found in any home. He wanted to sell his tractors. They sold for £5 and were purchased by notables such as George Washington and Chief Justice Oliver Ellsworth.[28]

The practitioner, or the patient himself if he desired, was instructed to stroke the affected part of the body with the Perkins' Patented Metallic Tractor rods to draw out the excess electrical energy. The instructions were to hold one of the tractors in each hand and stroke them over the area to be treated to extract pain. As the practitioner drew the rods downward over the afflicted area towards the patient's extremities, the pain was pulled supposedly downwards with them and finally out of the body. Specific manipulations varied with the disease to be removed. Perkins recommended their use for rheumatism, gout, and pleurisy. He later added treatments for paralysis, lameness, and deformities. Patients were advised to use the tractors for twenty minutes a day.

The curious part of the whole story is that Elisha Perkins was not a crank or quack, and he appears to have been genuine in his belief that the devices worked. He was a well-respected surgeon who had been educated at Yale, and was one of the founders of the Connecticut Medical Society. Perkins firmly believed that his metallic tractors were based on the latest theories of electricity and would cure pains in the head, face, teeth, chest, stomach, and back, as well as rheumatism and all joint pains.

The sale of tractors spread to Europe, including such countries as Denmark and Germany. They sold so well that Elisha's son, Benjamin D. Perkins, opened an office in London where he capitalized on the demand. A pair of tractors sold for £5 to physicians and £10 for general public.[29] The fad for using tractors eventually passed, but not until after thousands had been sold.[30]

The entire concept was eventually called into question after Dr. John Haygarth in England constructed similar tractors from wood. Experiments with five patients produced the same results as the metallic tractors. In 1800 Haygarth published the results of his study, questioning the effectiveness of the device, and concluding that the results were psychosomatic.[31]

Back in the United States, several disbelieving physicians also made tractors from lead, slate, wood, bone, and other materials, and found that they worked as well as Perkins' metallic version, indicating that non-conductors of electricity worked just as well as the metallic versions.[32] After reports of these findings were publicized, sales dropped and faith in the devices was lost.

The Connecticut Medical Society then became suspicious. They were able to duplicate the wooden tractor results, and in 1796 expelled Perkins from the society as a fraud.[33] Perkins went to New York City to offer his assistance during a yellow fever epidemic, but succumbed to the disease in 1799.

New Teeth from Old

Dentistry in the early 1800s was primitive at best and the limited dental care that was available consisted primarily of extracting bad teeth. The two choices for a man or woman with a toothache were to do nothing and put up with the pain, or to try to find a dentist and have the tooth pulled. If a person was in agony from an aching tooth and no dentist was available, in desperation he or she might go to the local blacksmith, who had pliers and pincers that could be used to perform an extraction.

If a tooth was not excessively decayed, a dentist might be able to drill out the cavity and insert a filling made from gold foil or tinfoil, held in place by creosote. An amalgam of silver, tin, and mercury was later used for fillings.

After decayed teeth were pulled out, replacement teeth were important, both for cosmetic reasons and to restore lost function. Early tooth replacements were made from carved bone, ivory, or even from natural animal or human teeth. Some early false teeth were fashioned from hippopotamus or elephant tusks. A set of false teeth cost about $8.

Some of the first false teeth in England were called "Waterloo Teeth." These were real human teeth from dead bodies, supposedly extracted from and named after the victims of the Battle of Waterloo. Others came from bodies dug up by grave-robbers or "resurrection men," who sold them to unsavory buyers. To make dentures, these real teeth were glued into hand-carved pieces of ivory from hippopotamus jaws. The result was that the "gums" were bone-white in color, which looked somewhat odd, but was better than having no teeth at all. Unfortunately these false teeth decayed like normal teeth and did not last long before having to be replaced.[34]

Before modern techniques for installing dentures were developed, false teeth were often simply glued to the remaining roots of the patient's own teeth. This procedure, however, was not particularly successful either. The remaining root of the tooth continued to decay in the jaw and the glue that was used soon discolored or turned black. With continued improvement of dental techniques, dentists learned how to extract the entire tooth in order to prevent further decay of the roots.

The development of the vulcanization of natural rubber by Charles Goodyear in 1839 led to the use of vulcanite (hard rubber) for dentures.[35] Dentists, noting the use of celluloid (a plastic based on cellulose nitrate) for billiard balls by J. Smith Hyatt in 1869, quickly adapted the same material for dentures.

The second half of the nineteenth century saw the development of improved false teeth that were made from porcelain, which was a mixture of the minerals feldspar, quartz, and clay, baked at high temperature to form a hard, impervious material that was ideal for dentures.

The Eudiometer

One of the serious problems in London in the mid–1800s was the massive amount of sewage that was created in the city every day and which ended up in the River Thames. Before a proper central sewer system was created for the city in 1858, upper-class homes had individual water closets and their own septic pits. The lower classes used outside privies or one in the cellar that was often just a wooden seat over a hole in the ground. Chamber pots for overnight use were often emptied out of the bedroom window into the street below. This practice was so common in the crowded and unsanitary streets of Edinburgh in Scotland that being unexpectedly showered from several stories above by the contents of a emptied chamber pot was known as an "Edinburgh baptism." The person tossing out the waste was supposed to call out the warning "gardyloo," from the French "*Gardez l'eau!*" meaning "Watch out for the water!" But often they didn't bother.

In London so much sewage overflowed the streets from all these inadequate arrangements that an appalling smell hung over the streets of the city. It became so bad that 1858 was known in London as the year of the "Great Stink." Sewage that had been flushed into the Thames floated downriver to Greenwich when the tide went out, then floated back up again when the tide came in. The air in the Houses of Parliament was so polluted with the smell of sewage that all the curtains were closed and soaked in chloride of lime to try to absorb the smell.[36]

Worried about death and disease, Victorian scientists measured the smelliness of the atmosphere with a device called a eudiometer, an instrument that was used to analyze gases by measuring the change in volume of a gas mixture that followed a physical change. Scientists used a version of the eudiometer that was developed by Alessandro Volta, the Italian physicist well known for his contributions to the development of the electric battery. Volta invented the eudiometer in 1777 for the purpose of testing the "goodness" of air, analyzing the flammability of gases, and to demonstrate the chemical effects of electricity. The device was perfect for the purpose as Volta's initial use of this instrument was for the study of smelly swamp gases (methane).

Operation of the device was quite simple. A long glass tube that was closed at the top was filled with oxygen and the gas being tested, in this case the polluted London atmosphere. The mixture was sealed into the tube with a cork. A spark was introduced into the gas chamber and, if the gases were flammable, they would explode and change the volume of gas within the test chamber. Measurements of the before and after volumes of gas was related to the "purity" or "goodness" of the air.

Needles, Probes and the Resuscitator

Acupuncture, the practice of inserting thin needles into the skin at different locations in the body to relieve pain and to cure ailments, has been a part of Chinese medicine for possibly as long as 7000 years. The insertion points did not necessarily reflect the specific site of the pain or affliction, but were locations along body channels called meridians, where Chinese doctors believed that life force energy flowed.

The Western medical profession was aware of acupuncture as far back as the 1700s and the technique was in use in England in the 1820s for the treatment of rheumatism. The needles used, however, were ordinary sewing needles. Some patients had an understandable reluctance to have these large needles forced into their flesh and unskilled practitioners often caused more pain than they relieved. Another hazard associated with the use of needles before the understanding of antiseptic conditions was the danger of introducing infection when piercing the skin. By the 1860s the practice had mostly fallen into disuse. Discredit for acupuncture also arose due to charlatans who offered cures for "male weaknesses," such as erectile dysfunction, premature ejaculation, and nocturnal emissions, by forcing needles into the perineum (the area between the genitals and the anus), the anal area, and even into the prostate.[37]

The use of acupuncture still appeared in William Osler's classic medical text *The Principles and Practice of Medicine* in the 1890s. His recommended method was to drive three and four-inch needles deep into the site of the pain, a technique which often caused more agony and rejection by the patient than it produced a cure. Luckily for the patient, Osler did recommend sterilizing the needles before use.

A renewed interest in acupuncture in Western medicine arose in the 1970s with the re-opening of diplomatic relations between China and the United States, and the popular fascination of the public with the new idea of needling. Some acupuncture research has been promising, but mostly inconclusive. Discussion and debate about the effectiveness of acupuncture still continues. Scientific evaluation has been mixed and scientists have found no definite mechanism to explain its effectiveness, which is important for scientific proof. There is no agreement on the mechanism by which it works, and some think the results are obtained via the placebo effect.[38]

A curious earlier offshoot of acupuncture and the use of needles was developed by a businessman named Carl Baunscheidt when he noted in 1848 that after several gnats landed on his hand and bit him, the pain of arthritis in his hand disappeared.[39] Accordingly, Baunscheidt developed a formal method of puncturing the skin called Baunscheidtism, using a device that he likened to a mechanical gnat for treatment by "counterirritation."[40]

The working part of the device consisted of a hollow cylinder, two inches deep and three inches in diameter, made of ebony or wood, and attached to a hollow tube that formed the handle of the mechanism. The cylinder contained thirty sharp needles about two inches long. The entire instrument was about twelve inches long. For

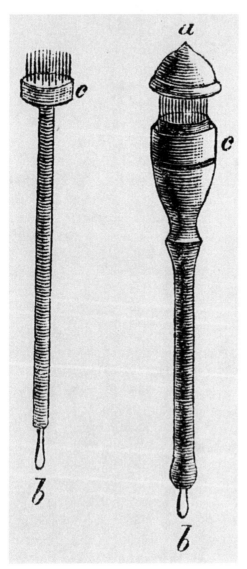

This is the *Lebenswecker* or "Life Awakener" that was used in an attempt to stimulate the newly-deceased to determine if life was still present. Thirty sharp two-inch needles were driven into the skin to try to elicit a reaction from a corpse. If there was no reaction to this extreme stimulation, the person was considered to be truly deceased. The sketch on the left shows the internal mechanism with the needles exposed; the picture on the right shows the assembled unit with a protective cap on the top (National Library of Medicine).

use, the operator pulled on a cord at the back of the mechanism that retracted the needles into the cylinder. He then placed the end of the cylinder over the affected area. When he released the cord, an internal spring in the handle forced the needles to shoot out again and penetrate the skin, making punctures in it to supposedly allow the release of any pathogenic substances trapped in the body.

Baunscheidt assumed that when the insects had bitten him, they had at the same time injected some substance that assisted in the healing process. So he developed an irritating oil with the magnificent name of "*Oleum Baunscheidti*" (Oil of Baunscheidt) that was applied with a chicken feather to the puncture wounds to assist in the healing. If the first treatment did not work, it was supposed to be repeated every ten days until the patient fully recovered.

Baunscheidt named his device the *Lebenswecker* (German for "Life Awakener"); in English it was named the Resuscitator. The Resuscitator was applied to the lower back to treat jaundice, to the abdomen for diarrhea, to the shoulder blades for malaria, behind the ears to cure baldness, and to the groin to cure chronic masturbation. The *Lebenswecker* was commonly used from 1851 until about 1915. Similar devices were made and sold by several other companies.

Premature Burial

The name for Baunscheidt's device is curious, but was probably because it had more to do with death than life. A secondary use for the Resuscitator was as a device to apply to the newly-deceased to avoid premature burial.

The Victorians were a particularly morbid society and were obsessed with death and disease, in part because they were surrounded by both in their daily lives. Mortality in Victorian times was high, due to a lack of knowledge of the cause of diseases that were incurable at the time, such as tuberculosis, cholera, typhoid, and diphtheria. One issue that terrified the living was that doctors at the time were not sure how to accurately determine that a patient was truly dead.

In 1819 the Doctor Regent of the Paris Faculty of Medicine wrote that one-third or perhaps even one-half of those who died in their beds were not actually dead when they were buried, and the "corpse" had merely been unconscious.[41] Such large numbers seem unlikely, but according to doctors of the nineteenth century this happened with some frequency.

Conditions that resembled death, such as being in a coma resulting from various diseases or accidents, respiratory collapse due to various poisonous gases, or the result of shocks from the new technology of electricity, were not uncommon. Thus the fear of being misdiagnosed and buried prematurely was widespread. Concerns were heightened because embalming was not a common practice until the time of the American Civil War, when it was used to preserve the bodies of soldiers who died far from home so that their remains could be shipped back to their families.

Nothing could equal the fear of the thought of being buried alive. Dreadful stories were told of disinterred coffins found with scratch marks on the underside of the lids where the "dead person" had tried to claw his or her way out. Whether true or not, the fears of the public were real.

To try to stimulate a response from the apparently dead, doctors would stick objects down the body's throat, tickle it with a feather, or blare a trumpet into its ear. The Resuscitator was promoted as one such instrument to apply to the newly-deceased to try to elicit a reaction to avoid premature burial. Being jabbed by thirty sharp, two-inch-long needles would presumably evoke some sort of response from those who were inert, but still among the living.

Auriculotherapy

Auriculotherapy, also referred to as auricular therapy, is a form of acupuncture treatment based on the idea that the outer portion of the ear (the pinna or auricle) has pressure points contained in its surface that mirror the parts of the body and contain connections to the entire body. The original therapy, called ear acupuncture, auricular acupuncture, or auriculoacupuncture, dated back to ancient China and involved the insertion of acupuncture needles into the outer ear. The theory was that conditions affecting the physical or mental health of the patient could be treated by stimulation of the pressure points on the surface of the ear.

Practitioners also said that electrical stimulation, acupuncture, or simple pressure on the appropriate points on the surface of the ear (a technique also known as acupressure) could lead to a dramatic decrease in pain in the corresponding body part. These mappings were not based on any medical findings or supported by any scientific evidence, and were therefore considered to be pseudo-science. There are no known anatomical pathways that connect the ear to the rest of the body.

Whether or not this approach works is currently still a matter of controversy. One controlled crossover study of thirty-six patients failed to find any difference in the method, and the study concluded that auriculotherapy was not an effective therapeutic procedure for chronic pain.[42] On the other hand, in another paper, two physicians who reviewed the scientific data related to auriculotherapy concluded that auriculotherapy was useful, particularly for addressing pain. Their review said that it was no longer possible to doubt the reality of the acupoints, and they claimed that clinical findings and experimentally reproducible data demonstrated the objective reality of the procedures.[43]

It's All in Your Head

Phrenology was the "science" of evaluating an individual's personality, intelligence, and character by examining the contours of his or her head. Phrenology claimed to explain why we behave the way we do, and how to develop desirable traits to become a better person.

Phrenology experts claimed that the human brain was composed of different organs, or regions, each of which was responsible for a specific mental or emotional trait. This was not a totally new thought as the idea that different parts of the brain controlled different bodily functions was put forward as far back as the time of Hippocrates. The degree of development of each trait in an individual's personality was theorized to be directly related to the degree of development, or actual size, of the corresponding organ in the brain. The skull, with its bumps and recesses, was presumed to reflect the shape of the underlying brain, thus an individual's character could be analyzed by the phrenologist through an examination of the size of the bumps on the subject's head.[44]

Phrenology had its origins in the 1790s when physician Franz Joseph Gall in Austria developed a system to assign intellectual ability and personality traits to specific regions of the head. He developed the theory that parts of the brain that were better developed than others tended to have larger bumps on the outside of the head. He further theorized that different parts of the brain controlled different functions and that the external shape of the skull corresponded to the shape of the particular brain underneath it. Thus he felt that studying bumps on the outside of the head would reveal which parts of the brain were better developed than others. The personality of the individual could then be categorized by the bumps. A large bump would be dominant in that person's characteristics.[45] For example, Gall theorized that thieves tended to have large bumps behind their ears.[46]

Gall studied hundreds of heads and concluded that there were twenty-seven inborn human characteristics. He did admit that not all of them were good ones, and in some individuals included tendencies towards theft and murder. Gall lectured extensively on the subject in Europe in the early 1800s, entertaining audiences as he traveled. Though Gall considered himself to be a serious scientist, he attracted people to his medicine-show type of lectures with music, drama, and other theatrics, such as exhibiting his large collection of skulls.

In 1804 Gall started a collaboration with German physician Johann Spurzheim. It was Spurzheim who named their work "phrenology," from the Greek words *phren* (for "mind") and *ology* ("the study of").[47] Gall and Spurzheim later parted professional company after they disagreed on the purpose and methodology of their work.

Though Spurzheim was not the first to promote phrenology in the United States, he helped to popularize the concept on a lecture tour of New England in 1832. His talks were very popular because he presented the idea that anyone could develop desirable qualities in themselves through personal initiative and perseverance. This concept fit well with the American dream that no matter what a person's origins, he or she could improve themselves into the type of person they wanted to be and achieve their desired goals.

The idea that a person could use science to solve their personality problems was popular among the general public. The working classes, in particular, were attracted to the idea because it gave them hope for advancement through self-improvement. Unfortunately Spurzheim caught a cold after his tour and died a short time later. Ironically, his own skull became part of a phrenological collection at the Boston Phrenological Society.[48]

In the wake of Spurzheim's success, two brothers, Lorenzo Niles Fowler and Orson Squire Fowler, were responsible for promoting and commercializing phrenology in the United States in the 1830s. Though they were self-taught students of phrenology, their tireless efforts made them America's most renowned bump experts, as they promoted the idea that phrenology could determine a person's characteristics which could in turn lead to social and moral reform that would benefit mankind. And they conveniently happened to sell whatever was needed to make this happen, including charts, books, models of the organs of the brain, and ways to interpret the measurements.

They also had a shrewd sense of business and a flair for the theatrical. They appeared in theaters and lecture halls across the eastern United States in 1834 where they explained the basics of phrenology and offered phrenological examinations to determine the personality traits of attendees. The examiner felt the bumps on each person's head and recorded their size in each region. The results were then correlated to a chart that revealed the personality traits. The lecture was free, but the measurements and categorization of personality was not.

The mental factors and traits supposedly revealed by the bumps covered such characteristics as sublimity (#21b, love of grandeur), acquisitiveness (#9, accumulation and frugality), ailimentiveness (#8, appetite, hunger, love of food), agreeableness (#37d, suavity, pleasantness), amativeness (#1, sexual and connubial love), adhesiveness (#3, friendship, sociability), inhabitiveness (#4, love of home) and the grandly named philoprogenitiveness (#2, parental love).[49] The Fowlers' literature contained a detailed explanation of each of the characteristics and what the size of each bump meant in terms of the individual's personality.

The Fowler brothers promoted phrenology with vast amounts of literature. In 1835 they founded a publishing house with their brother-in-law Samuel Wells to publish a comprehensives series of

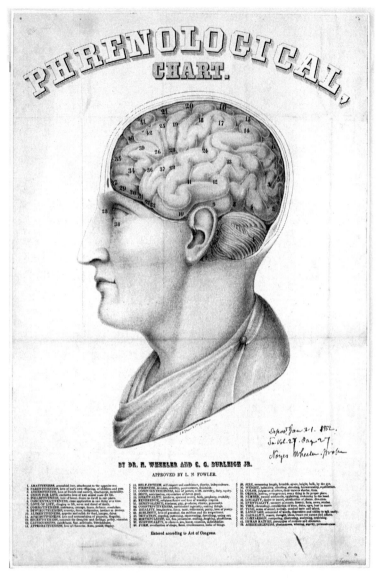

This phrenological chart, approved by expert Lorenzo Fowler himself, lists various personality characteristics by number and then links them to the areas of the brain to which they supposedly corresponded. Phrenologists made measurements of a subject's head and then characterized the individual according to the prominence of various bumps. Popular with the public were phrenological readings to obtain information on vocational guidance, employment counseling, and suitable marriage prospects. Phrenology was popular in the United States from the 1830s until the early 1900s (Library of Congress).

books on phrenology, physiology, temperance, and a wide variety of other contemporary health and reform topics. Fowler & Wells was one of the country's largest publishing houses at the time, and became the leading publisher of phrenology books. In 1838 they started publishing the *American Phrenological Journal.* Both Orson and Lorenzo Fowler were part of the faculty at the New York Hygeio-Therapeutic College and lectured extensively on phrenology in the 1850s.[50]

The Fowlers' New York City offices became known as the Phrenological Cabinet. A "cabinet" was a type of museum containing notable collections of varied objects related to natural history. The term originally described a room rather than today's description of a piece of furniture. The Fowlers' cabinet was essentially a museum of curiosities related to phrenology, including the heads of murderers and pirates, casts of skulls, and similar peculiarities from around the world. Various skulls were used to demonstrate examples of a person's character traits.

Although the Fowlers were the most prominent in the field, other practitioners promoted phrenology and traveled around the country performing head examinations and offering personality readings. At phrenology's height, one estimate was that there were more than 20,000 itinerant phrenologists.[51]

Many Americans consulted phrenologists to assess the size and shape of their heads in order to understand their personality and mental abilities. Traveling phrenologists tended to concentrate their public readings on career pathways or how to identify suitable marriage prospects, rather than on science. A popular theme with the public was vocational guidance and employment counseling. If a person knew the line of work he or she wished to pursue, that individual could then work to cultivate the brain faculties necessary for success in that field. Advice on love and finding a suitable husband or wife concentrated on using phrenological charts to help customers find congenial life companions. Phrenologists advised parents on how to raise children based on head shape and size to take best advantage of their offsprings' characteristics.

To perform the actual measurement of the head, the Fowlers used a device called a craniometer, a caliper-like device that measured the bumps. When rotated over the skull, the device produced a series of measurements that could be compared to a phrenological chart to determine the characteristics of the person. A reading of the head took from thirty to sixty minutes. The results tended to be flattering. Any bad tendencies were usually couched in vague terms so as not to offend the customer.

Even though phrenology was falling from its peak in popularity in the early 1900s, in 1905 Henry C. Lavery of Superior, Wisconsin, developed a complicated looking device called the Psychograph to mechanize the tedious process of measuring the bumps and contours of a person's head. Based on the measurements it made, the machine then printed out an analysis and assessment of the person's characteristics and personality.[52] The information could be correlated to a chart to determine a suitable vocation for the subject and hopefully find a job for which they were well-suited. The machine was a popular novelty attraction (and moneymaker!) in theater lobbies, department stores, and local fairs.

The Psychograph offered a time-saving for the operator. A traditional phrenologist took up to an hour to "read" the head manually, while the machine could produce results in about five minutes. The operator placed a headpiece that looked somewhat like an old-fashioned hair dryer over the top of the head. This allowed multiple thin rods with blunt ends to make contact with the surface of the head. How far the rods projected from their individual holders when they made contact with the head determined the readings. The probe readings were matched to evaluations stored inside the machine, which then printed out thirty-two personality characteristics on a scale of one to five that corresponded to from "deficient" (poor) to "very superior" (excellent).

The Psychograph did not measure brain waves, or any other brain-related artifact, but only the physical size of the head and its contours. As the readings were based on the size of the head, people with large heads naturally received high scores. In fact, as author Bob McCoy has correctly observed, measurements from a large watermelon could turn out to have the characteristics of a highly intelligent individual.[53]

Only about forty Psychographs were built. Though never widespread, the machine was used into the 1920s, then faded away in the 1930s. The machines leased for $35 a month with a $2,000 down payment.

By the early 1900s phrenology was losing its scientific status and even its popular appeal. Interpreting human characteristics by the shape of the skull had been popular among the water-cure practitioners

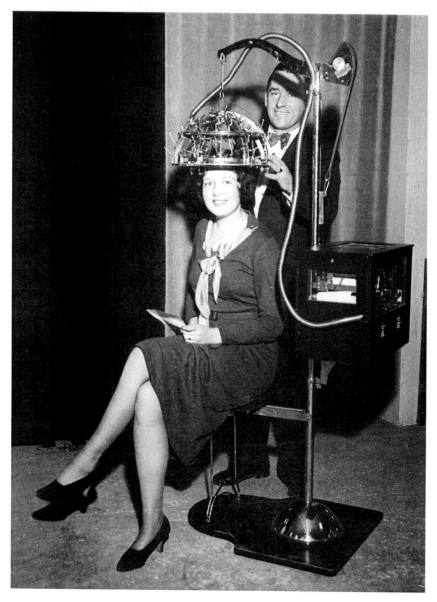

Photographed in 1931, this woman is demonstrating the use of the Psychograph, a phrenology machine used for automatically measuring the bumps and contours on her head. This complicated-looking device was developed in 1905 by Henry C. Lavery of Superior, Wisconsin, to mechanize the process of measuring a person's head for phrenological analysis. Based on the measurements, the machine then printed out an analysis and assessment of the person's characteristics and personality (Library of Congress).

of the mid–1800s, but was later discredited and largely abandoned by the beginning of the 1900s when medical science offered better tools for understanding the brain.[54] As the specialty of neuroscience evolved, scientists discovered that areas of the brain that determined characteristics, such as speech and vision, were not located where the phrenologists had indicated.

By the early twentieth-century phrenology had fallen into disuse.

FIVE

Magnetic Devices

Several hundred years ago, electricity and magnetism were considered to be two separate forces of nature. Both were used for treating illness. Electricity was used to send an electrical current through the skin that was thought to replace vital bodily energy. Magnets were used for treatment because they radiated an unseen mysterious field that was thought to have curative powers. The two are now known to be fundamentally interlinked as a consequence of Einstein's theory of special relativity, and magnetism is just one aspect of the combined phenomenon of electromagnetism.

After discovering that lodestone, a black mineral that contains a form of magnetite (a magnetic iron ore), attracted pieces of iron and steel, the ability of magnetism to influence and move objects remotely without directly touching them seemed like a mysterious power. For this reason, magnetic lodestone was thought to possibly be the "philosopher's stone," the legendary substance that was capable of turning base metals, such as mercury, into gold. The philosopher's stone was also reputed to be useful for reversing the aging process and lengthening the span of human life.

Pondering the uncanny natural ability of lodestone to attract iron objects without touching them, alchemists wondered if this mysterious mineral might have other useful properties that could be used to influence or cure illness remotely from outside the body. Accordingly, during the Middle Ages, physicians performed experiments to see if lodestone might be able to cure or influence such diverse ailments as epilepsy, gout, arthritis, baldness, diarrhea, bleeding, and other common medical problems of the time. In the early 1500s Swiss scientist, physician, and alchemist Paracelsus (Philippus von

Hohenheim) attributed occult powers to lodestone and used it to treat epilepsy.

Animal Magnetism

In the 1800s there was a strong belief that the human body was energized by a mysterious vital force. Healers had tried to explain the workings of this "vital force" or "nervous energy" for a long time, but the explanations were always nebulous. When magnetism was discovered, however, the belief in a magnetic fluid within the body grew and healers thought that by realigning a patient's internal magnetic field they could improve overall health.

Physician H.H. Sherwood, for example, wrote *A Manual for Magnetizing* in 1845. He claimed that the body was a magnet and disease occurred when the body's magnetic forces were not in equilibrium. To counteract this he developed a "magnetic machine" that he used to treat disease. Though still categorized as a magnetic device at the time, the machine actually generated electricity. It consisted of a wheel driven by a crank that rotated an armature to generate sparks. This sent an electric current (and shocks) to brass cylinders held by the patient in each hand. A later version of the machine used a wet-cell battery to generate electricity.

Magnetic Devices

The literature on magnetism and electricity increased steadily between 1835 and 1855. One of earliest publications on the subject was *Manual of Magnetism* (1842) by Daniel Davis. The book provided a complete analysis of magnets and electromagnets, and included Davis' catalog of various types of apparatus that he sold for medical use. Davis later wrote *Medical Applications of Electricity* (1846).

After the American Civil War, magnetic medicine became popular as an alternative form of treatment, and the concept of magnetic healing stimulated the development of a large array of questionable medical devices. Treatments involving magnetic devices were claimed to improve physical strength, stamina, and resistance to disease. The use of magnets was supposed to help treat a wide variety of physical ailments, including arthritis, asthma, headaches, writer's cramp, gout, varicose veins, insomnia, stress, sore muscles, cancer, warts, and problems of the kidneys, liver, lungs, stomach, and bowels.

Devices for magnetic treatment quickly appeared in the form of belts, bracelets, shoe insoles, and mattresses to relieve stress and improve blood circulation. Manufacturers also promoted magnetic seat cushions, magnetic coils, bandages, and adhesive patches. Wearable magnetic devices included body pads, knee braces, mittens, back braces, eye masks, thigh supporters, elbow supporters, wrist bands, ankle wraps, and back supporters.

Magnetic corsets that incorporated a series of small magnets in the material were popular among women. One 1885 advertisement for Harness' Magnetic Corsets from the Medical Battery Company of London said, "By wearing this Perfectly designed Corset the most awkward figure becomes graceful and elegant, the internal organs are speedily strengthened. The chest is aided in its healthy development. And the entire system is invigorated."

Dr. Chester I. Thatcher of the Chicago Magnetic Shield Company promoted a series of clothes in the 1880s to enhance the magnetic field of the human body. Thatcher's hypothesis was that the iron content of the blood made it a conductor of magnetism inside the body. He theorized that if this iron did not absorb adequate magnetic power from the atmosphere, then disease would occur. His solution to the problem was to provide ways that he thought would improve this condition.

Thatcher claimed that his magnetic shields would heal any disease that afflicted the human race. In describing the product line, Thatcher advertised, "…magnetism is radiated from the Lung Shield, Belt and Lower Leggings into all the vital organs, as well as lower extremities, giving new life and activity to the circulation from head to foot, thus strengthening all the vital organs and large nerve centers, and assisting nature in the work of eliminating diseased conditions by reason of the better circulation of the blood that is established as soon as the Shields are applied." He also claimed, "This set of shields contains over eight hundred powerful Magnetic Storage Batteries that are guaranteed to hold their power." One of his newspaper advertisements was

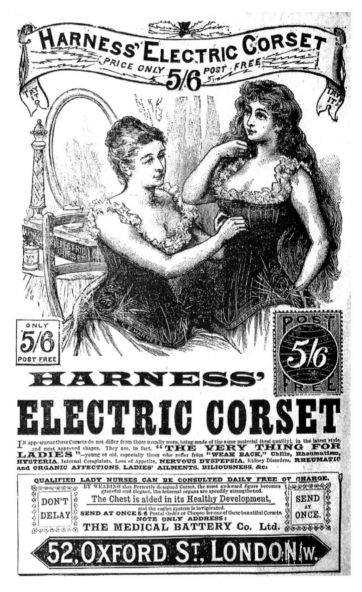

Though this advertisement from the Medical Battery Company of London is for Harness' Electric Corset, this was in reality a magnetic corset as it incorporated a series of small magnets in the material. Note the symbolic little lightning flashes coming from each of the women's hips to denote the power of the garment. Perfect for everyday use, magnetic corsets were popular among women as they offered the promise of continuous treatment while being worn, and were claimed to improve physical strength, stamina, and resistance to disease (author's collection).

accompanied by an illustration showing a man surrounded by powerful magnetic lines of force radiating from his torso and legs, and lightning bolts stabbing out from his feet.

As one of Thatcher's premier products, his advertisements promoted his Magnetic Belt for lame back, weakness of the spine, and all diseases of the kidneys. For men, the belt looked like a supporter that strapped around the lower abdomen. For women it was expanded upwards into a garment that covered the torso from the shoulders, over the bust, and down to the hips, looking like an old-fashioned corset. He claimed that his belt was so powerful that it would provide relief from back pain within five minutes. He somewhat immodestly claimed, "It is the crowning triumph of the nineteenth century!" He also took a jab at his competition with, "Do not compare the Belt with the bogus trash advertised as Electric, etc." His belts were advertised to contain "Over 100 magnetic batteries, distributing their soothing power to the abdominal organs and muscles."[1]

Thatcher's Magnetic Kidney belt was similar to the men's magnetic belt, but was designed to sit higher on the hips. As well as the kidneys, it was claimed to also treat indigestion, aches and pains, and inactive bowels. Thatcher's Magnetic Foot Batteries, which were actually shoe insoles, were claimed to keep the feet warm in cold weather by increasing the circulation of blood. They sold for $1 a pair or three pairs for $2. He believed so strongly in his own products that he commonly wore a magnetic cap, vest, sock liners, and shoe insoles. He felt that by doing so he was restoring the "harmonious vibrations of the brain." Not everybody agreed and, like many other promoters of quack medical claims, Thatcher felt that the traditional medical community was conspiring against him, rather than supporting him.

In the 1920s Professor Charles Bidwell of Chicago also manufactured an extensive line of clothing items that was intended for magnetic healing. His magnetic caps were recommended for neuralgia (severe pain associated with a nerve), poor memory, weak eyes, dizziness, and all types of headache. He made throat shields to prevent hoarseness and sore throats. His lung protectors were used for pain in the chest, heart trouble, weak lungs, and pneumonia. Belts for gentlemen were used to treat backache, and provide sure relief for kidney, liver, and bowel problems. Equivalent belts for the ladies offered relief for kidney troubles and all female pelvic suffering. Magnetic insoles were used for leg aches and cold feet. When the insoles were used with Bidwell's sleeping cap they could supposedly cure insomnia.[2] The rationale for Bidwell's magnetic clothing was, "They set up vital action in all the organs, tissues and great nerve centers, giving warmth, protection, action and life; removing all aches, pains, weaknesses and nervous languor."[3]

Magnetic chains, in the form of a necklace, such as Dr. Raphael's Famous Electro-Magnetic Chains, were (and still are) sold for the relief of pain.

Mesmerism

One of the more convoluted, but best publicized, methods of magnetic healing involved a controversial physician by the name of Franz Mesmer. Mesmer believed that the body was composed primarily of some sort of magnetic fluid. He developed a treatment method called mesmerism, a pseudo-science that purportedly healed by freeing and redirecting energy fields in the human body, using magnets to realign the patient's internal energy fields. The basic concept was that in illness the flow of internal energy was blocked within the body, but that it could be manipulated by an external magnetic force and released to produce improved health.[4]

Franz Anton Mesmer was born in Germany and received a medical degree from the University of Vienna in 1766. In his doctoral dissertation Mesmer proposed that the gravitational pull of the sun, moon, and planets affected human health through a universal force that influenced an invisible magnetic fluid within the human body. Mesmer proposed that the nervous fluids in the body were subject to the universe's invisible gravitational forces, just like the tides. He based his theory on ideas that went back to the sixteenth century and Paracelsus. The concepts of nervous fluids circulating in the body went back even further to the Roman physician Galen, who thought that the body contained animal spirits that flowed through the nerves.

Eventually Mesmer came to believe that disruptions to the flow of the nervous magnetic fluid caused disease. He knew that magnets could affect metal objects without direct contact, thus he reasoned that magnets might be able to affect illness by magnetic fields acting inside the body. He believed that a physician could re-direct the flow of nervous fluid from outside the body and theorized that disease might thus be controlled by magnets, since magnetism could control other physical entities without actual physical contact.

Mesmer was a well-established practitioner in Vienna in the 1770s when he attempted to treat patients through "animal magnetism," an idea that he adapted from Professor Maximillian Hell, a Jesuit priest and astronomer at the University of Vienna. Hell had applied magnets to the bodies of patients to treat painful muscle conditions with some seeming success.[5]

Mesmer started treating patients in a magnetized environment. To counteract the disruptions that he thought were present within the body, he developed magnetized sheets, magnetized water for bathing, magnetized plates and eating utensils, and magnetized clothing.

By moving magnets over a patient's body, Mesmer thought that he could cure imbalances or misalignments of the force field by manipulating the fluid in the afflicted area and thus make the patient feel better. Later he came to believe that gifted healers (such as himself, naturally) could do the same by simply moving their hands over the patient's body. Mesmer's theories contained just enough science to be believable. His hypothesis of a magnetic fluid was derived from the contemporary theories of electromagnetism and the ether.[6]

Mesmer's initial success came in 1774, when he treated a female patient named Francisca Österlin, who was beset by recurrent attacks of hysteria and periodic seizures, accompanied by symptoms of vomiting, fainting, temporary blindness, and paralysis. When Mesmer placed magnets on her abdomen and legs, she reported feeling a sensation of fluid running through her body and, after several treatments, claimed to be cured.[7] Mesmer was encouraged enough to proceed.[8]

Mesmer continued to experiment and found that wooden and other non-magnetic devices could achieve the same results, but only if used by him. As he continued to give treatments, he believed that he could influence the body's internal forces simply by moving his hands over the patient without using magnets. Thus he reasoned that if varied objects could affect the nervous fluid, it must be the power of the healer that produced the cure, rather than the magnets.

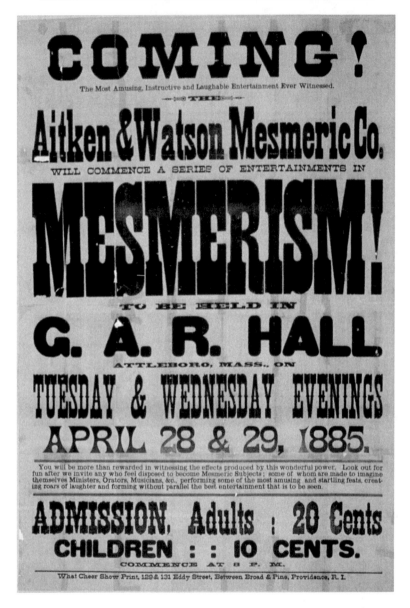

Mesmerism, named after physician Franz Mesmer, was a controversial practice that was frowned on by the conventional medical establishment after accusations of impropriety with his patients. Nevertheless, mesmerism was adopted by some magnetic healers, though it was never accepted by mainstream science. The practice also degenerated into a sideshow attraction practiced by itinerant showmen, as advertised in this handbill for a demonstration in Attleboro, Massachusetts, in 1885 (Library of Congress).

Mesmer treated cases of vomiting, toothaches, blindness, paralysis, urinary retention, and depression, but his methods were criticized by his peers. Some patients reported that their symptoms were cured, which may have had a psychosomatic basis. Many, however, were no better after treatment. Mesmer became discredited in Vienna when controversy arose after he treated a blind patient named Maria Paradis, who possibly had psychosomatic vision problems. The public began to think of him as a fraud, so in 1778 he left Austria for France.

Mesmer started to treat patients in Paris with great success. He developed a magnetic instrument that he called a *baquet*, which in French means "tub" or "bucket." The device was a large, covered, circular wooden bucket, four feet in diameter and a foot deep. The tub held bottles of magnetized water arranged over a layer of magnetized glass and iron, with thin iron rods coming out of the top. The rods were pliable and long enough that they could be applied to specific body parts when treating patients. Mesmer had four of these magnetic tubs in his Paris treatment room.

The typical procedure was described by a British physician named MacKay. As many as twenty patients clustered around each *baquet* and were treated at the same time. Patients, primarily women, gathered around and held each other's hands and pressed their knees together to "allow the magnetic fluid to flow" from one to the other. Suitably solemn music was played on a piano in the corner of the room, because Mesmer felt that music helped to reinforce the flow of animal magnetism.[9]

Mesmer himself, dressed in long, flowing, lilac-colored robes, then entered the room and walked from patient to patient, staring deeply into the eyes of each one. As he did so, he touched or stroked each one with his hands or his foot-long iron "magnetic wand." He felt that because illness was a stoppage of the flow of magnetic fluid through the individual, he had to create a violent reaction to activate the body and re-establish its normal functioning. As he touched each individual, his goal was to make each one go into a frenzy of convulsions, hysterical laughter, screams, and fainting, which he called "the crisis."[10] Mesmer said, "The crisis is an effort of nature ... to disperse the obstacles which impede circulation, to dissolve and evacuate the molecules which form such obstructions...."[11]

Mesmer would then stroke the unconscious women's faces, breasts, spines, and abdomens with his magnetic wand until they returned to consciousness and recovered.[12] Mesmer's critics felt that the onset of the crisis stage after repeated stroking and fondling appeared to closely parallel sexual arousal and orgasm.[13]

Mesmer was assisted by a series of helpers, who were all handsome young men. Each of these assistant magnetizers seated himself in close proximity to a patient with their knees between his. Part of the treatment consisted of staring the patient fixedly in the eyes while rubbing the patient between the knees, massaging their spines, and applying gentle pressure to the breasts of the ladies while soft music played in the background. Eventually the cheeks of most of the women glowed and they suddenly went into convulsive fits, laughing, sobbing, and shrieking out loud as they did. Some even fainted. This was the "crisis" that Mesmer was trying to achieve.[14]

Although critics felt that Mesmer's procedure was questionable at the very least, Mesmer did not believe that he was a fraud. Mesmer estimated that he treated more than 8000 patients during his six years in Paris. Many patients went into hypnotic trances and felt better afterwards, and it appeared that he had discovered the power of hypnotism and suggestion.[15]

Conventional physicians, however, remained unimpressed with his magical force and in 1784 King Louis XVI appointed a scientific commission to evaluate Mesmer's claims. The members included electrical authority Benjamin Franklin, who was then the American ambassador to France, renowned chemist Antoine Lavoisier, and physician Joseph de Guillotin, the inventor of the guillotine.

After three months of investigation, the commission also remained unimpressed. They could not find any beneficial effects from the treatments, even after watching patients being treated and going through Mesmer's crisis stage. After suitable investigation they concluded that the invisible "magnetic fluid" did not exist and that the reactions and fainting had been due to other causes. They concluded that the convulsions during the crisis were due to suggestion and overly active imaginations on the part of susceptible patients.[16] The majority of Mesmer's patients were women and the investigating commission felt that they were more susceptible than men to suggestion. In hindsight, it would appear that they had been hypnotized (mesmerized).

Even though Mesmer denied any impropriety, gossip and the accusations of "outraging women" became too overwhelming. The discredited Mesmer left Paris and traveled through Europe. He finally relocated to Switzerland, where he died in 1815.

Though Mesmer left Paris, his following did not go away and mesmeric sessions continued to be held, even though there were concerns that women patients could be compromised by these activities.

Magnetic healing was introduced to America by Charles Poyen in 1835, who claimed to be able to heal rheumatism, liver disease, and other illnesses. Poyen called it animal magnetism. Others called it mesmerism, but also animal magnetism, electro-biology, etherology, mental electricity, pathetism, psycheism, psychodunamy, and therapeutic sarcognomy.[17]

Apparently determined not to be outdone, in the 1850s John Jacobus Flournoy of Georgia developed what he called Flournoy's Medical Headband, which combined and concentrated "the hidden virtues of Animal Magnetism, Mesmerism, Electrisity [*sic*], Magic and the Manifestation of the Spirits—together with impulses from the Aurora Borealis."[18] It must have been an awesome combination indeed.

Though mesmerism was used in America and was adopted by some magnetic healers, it was never accepted by mainstream science. Support and opposition for the concepts and practice continued to rage from various sides. Mesmerists typically continued to pass their hands over the patient's body, either in the air over the patient or by making direct contact. Some used Mesmer's magnetic wand.

Mesmerism continued to be popular in the United States through the 1930s for curing ailments from hysteria to elusive pain, and appeared to work at least for some of those afflictions that probably had a psychosomatic basis. The term "mesmerism" later acquired undesirable and occult overtones, as it was thought that a mesmerist could control the minds of others.[19]

Magnets Revived

Magnetic devices are still promoted for healing.[20] Various modes of action have been proposed to explain their action. Some of them are that magnets connect the user to the earth's magnetic field, that magnets align the elements in the body, that magnets dilate blood vessels and increase blood flow, that magnets alter the pH balance (acidity or alkalinity) of body fluids, and that magnets attract the iron in the blood and in this manner stimulate blood circulation.

Some devices that claimed to heal through magnetism were obvious frauds. For example, copper bracelets claimed to relieve arthritis, neuralgia (nerve pain), and general soreness cannot achieve these effects through magnetism, because copper does not have magnetic properties. The same is true of "magnetic combs" that are made from aluminum, which is also a non-magnetic material.

The 1990s saw a resurgence of interest in magnets for healing when major league baseball players started wearing magnets to improve their performance. In 1994 one company sold magnetic shoe insoles that had tiny magnets embedded in their surface, that were supposed to "ground" the user to the earth's magnetic field to prevent disease. They sold for $60.

Although magnet therapy continues to be used, the Food and Drug Administration has concluded that there is no scientific evidence that magnets have a permanent beneficial effect for the treatment of cancer, or for the relief of pain.[21]

SIX

The Mysteries of Electricity

The period between about 1860 and 1930 were the golden years of quackery. The beginning of this period coincided with the upswing of the age of technology. Electricity was finding practical applications, the country was slowly being electrified, electrical machines were rapidly being invented, and quack electrical devices started to proliferate. By the end of this period, government regulations and the Post Office had shut down most of the electrical quacks.

Electricity was regarded as a mysterious, unseen force and, before it was understood, was seen as a magical type of energy. The power of lightning, St. Elmo's Fire dancing on ship's rigging and sharp rocks at high altitude, and the blue flash and crackle of static electric discharges were seen as something beyond comprehension. During the Middle Ages frightened people thought that lightning was a manifestation of the wrath of God.[1] Thus, when scientists discovered how to create electricity in the laboratory and started to experiment with it, they were often accused of taking on the role of the supreme being and trying to control divine might. Electricity was seen as such a powerful and mysterious force that when Mary Shelley wrote her novel *Frankenstein, or the Modern Prometheus* in 1818, it was used as the essence of the life force that Baron Frankenstein used to bring his gruesome creation to life.

In the late nineteenth-century, popular culture was full of similar electrical fables, fads, follies, and fantasies. Electricity, for example, played a part in plots of some of the sensationalist dime novels. L. Frank Baum, who wrote the popular *Wizard of Oz* series of books, wrote stories such as "The Master Key: An Electrical Fairy Tale," in which a boy unleashed the Demon of Electricity from his electrical set.

Pseudo-scientific theories of health, combined with only a rudimentary understanding of electricity, made Victorians think that electricity was indeed the life force and that it could cure all physical ailments and improve poor health. As a treatment method it produced tangible results that the patient could see and feel. As a consequence, both legitimate and quack doctors used machines that generated electricity as the ultimate energy source and curing force. Medical quacks, of course, claimed that they could cure any disease with electricity.

How It All Began

The ancient Greeks observed that when the fossilized tree resin known as amber was rubbed with substances such as paper, feathers, or cloth, some mysterious force was created and the two materials were attracted to each other. These early scientists had unknowingly discovered static electricity and the principle that negative and positive charges attract. The name "electricity" was derived from the Greek word *electron* for amber.

Static electricity was one of the oldest forms of electrical treatment of the human body. Electricity was used in medicine by Aetius, a Greek physician of the sixth century, for example, who recommended the treatment of gout by standing on a torpedo fish, a type of electric stingray.[2] In another form of electric treatment, a fish that produced an electrical charge was wrapped around a patient's head to treat migraine headaches.

The scientific study of electricity as it related to living organisms started in 1780 when Italian physician and physicist Luigi Galvani, professor of anatomy at the University of Bologna, noted that the muscles in a frog's leg twitched when he applied static electricity to it. After observing this, he thought that he had found the source of animal vitality, naming the phenomenon (perhaps unfortunately) "animal electricity." He continued to experiment further with nerves and muscles, and tried to prove that electricity was the vital force that powered all biological actions.

Static electricity could be stored for short periods with the use of a Leyden jar. The Leyden jar, developed in 1745, was a glass, crock-like container with a conductive metallic coating on the outside of the jar and another on the inside, separated from each other by the glass of the jar. Static electricity was stored as positive and negative charges on the two metal coatings, separated by the electrically-insulating properties of the glass.

Alessandro Giuseppe Volta, professor of physics at the University of Pavia in Italy, subsequently showed that the source of Galvani's frog muscle contractions was due to an electrical voltage created when his dissecting tools, which were made from two dissimilar metals, came into contact with the muscle. The fluid in the frog's leg acted as a conductor between them. In other words, Galvani's metal tools combined with the frog's leg had created a primitive battery that activated the muscles.

Further experiments became possible after Volta discovered that he could generate electricity by combining two different metals, such as copper and zinc. He created the first practical battery in 1799, which consisted of a series of alternating discs of copper and zinc, separated by paper soaked in vinegar.[3]

The Leyden jar previously used to store static electricity was a somewhat erratic method that slowly self-discharged over time. Volta's discovery of the battery meant that scientists could now produce a supply of electricity when and where they wanted, and did not have to rely on the variable nature of static sparks.

Electricity as Nerve Force

After the discovery of the influence of electricity on the nervous system, many scientists and legitimate physicians experimented with electricity. As scientists studied these mysterious forces and animal experiments, along with the work of Galvani and Faraday, and built on previous knowledge about the action of electricity, some theorized that what had been earlier called the "vital force," "nervous fluid," "vital energy," or "nervous energy" of the body was the same as or similar to electricity.[4] The difference between magnetism and electricity as the vital force quickly became blurred.

Given this basis, electrical machines were seen as being capable of transferring energy directly into the nerves and muscles, thus increasing the body's energy reserves and forcing out disease. The application of low levels of electricity to muscles may have helped with minor pains, as indeed do today's Transcutaneous Electrical Nerve Stimulators (TENS) devices.

So popular was the concept of an electrical life force that the idea made its way into popular literature, such as the fictitious extraordinary energy life-force *Vril* that was supposedly pervasive in all nature in Edward Bulwer-Lytton's novel *The Coming Race*, published in 1871.

Static Electric Treatments

In the 1500s William Gilbert, physician to Queen Elizabeth I of England, promoted the use of static electricity for treatments after he noted that amber and sulfur when rubbed with wool, or glass rubbed with silk, developed a static electric charge, and produced a spark when touched to the skin. He treated muscle weakness, neuralgia, and skin conditions by conducting a spark to the particular part of the body with the ailment.[5] The static spark to the patient produced by the sudden release of electrical charge caused muscle contractions.

An early type of frictional machine to produce static electricity for use in treating muscular and nervous disorders was developed around 1662 by Otto von Guericke, a German scientist and inventor from Magdeburg. Jean-Martin Charcot, a French neurologist and professor of pathology, who followed Franz Mesmer in hypnotizing subjects, used static sparks at his clinic in Paris for the treatment of nervous disorders.[6]

Further understanding of the characteristics of electricity as applied to the body expanded in the eighteenth century. In 1788 Edward Nairne, a London instrument maker, constructed an electrostatic generator for medical use. The device produced static electricity through friction created between a revolving glass cylinder and a rod made of amber. The patient was insulated from the ground, and treatment consisted of drawing sparks from the body part being treated. Experiments with the device were apparently not particularly meaningful or successful.[7] But in 1820 one London clinic reported 4,000 patients were cured by electricity. In 1836 Guy's Hospital in London had a special "electrifying room."

In the late 1800s machines commonly used friction to produce static electricity. The electrical charge was produced by glass plates that rotated at high speed against small brushes and produced a static charge of very high voltage. To give this some perspective, about 25,000 volts of static electricity is required to produce a spark an inch long in dry air.[8]

One of the common machines used to generate static was named the Holtz machine, which was improved in 1883 by British inventor James Wimshurst, who designed the Wimshurst generator.[9] Wimshurst built more than ninety different machines to generate static electricity.[10] The basic method was that two large glass discs were placed close together and rotated in opposite directions by turning a crank. Brushes placed against the discs separated the positive and negative electrical charges, and stored them with a Leyden jar. When the jar was charged up and ready for use, one of the metallic coatings was electrically attached to the patient via a copper wire, and the other coating was attached to a metal probe. In this way the stored static electricity in the jar could be discharged into a particular part of the body. The resulting spark jumping to the skin produced a jolt for the patient, giving the sensation of a powerful electrical shock, one that is well-known to anyone who has scuffed their feet across a dry carpet then touched a metallic light switch and received a nasty surprise.

Static electricity was applied to patients from a static generator in the form of direct sparks, a static bath, a static breeze (called *soufflé*, or blowing), and Morton (static induction) current. For the "static bath" and the "static head breeze," the static charge was applied to the patient from an electrode close to the body, but without touching it and causing a spark to discharge. Static electricity was applied like this for treatment of nervous headaches, insomnia, and other nervous states.[11]

The first manual of electrotherapy was published in 1744 by German physician and engineer Christian Kratzenstein, who started experimenting with electrical charges to treat patients with such diverse ailments as rheumatism and plague.[12] He advocated electricity for the treatment of paralytics as early as 1745.[13]

In 1871 a German scientist named Steiner discovered that electric shocks were capable of reviving people after cardiac arrest.[14] He revived a patient who appeared to be dead by passing a weak electric current directly through his heart. Many people saw no difference between this type of application of new technology and magic, and believed that electricity could do anything.

One of the amateur tinkerers was Andrew Crosse from Somerset, England. In one of his experiments in 1836 he passed a current through a solution of powdered flint in acid. After two weeks he noticed that the solution contained a series of tiny insects or mites, similar to gnats. Unfortunately the newspapers got wind of this and publicized his experiment as the man who had made life with electricity, calling him a modern Frankenstein. Crosse denied that he had done anything of the kind, but the story was believed by a gullible public and simply confirmed the general feeling that electricity was the life force itself.[15]

Enthusiasm for medical electricity grew after the American Civil War in the mid–1860s. Due to the rebellion against Heroic Medicine and its lack of cures that worked, many people were willing to try something new. After the notion spread that the human body was powered by electricity, electrical treatments seemed like the logical next hope for a universal cure. After all, muscles and nerves had been shown to respond to electrical currents, therefore it seemed logical that electrical treatments should be able to infuse the body with energy. Patients were happy to sit in electric baths, or be electrified, or subject themselves to sparks of static electricity drawn from their bodies in the hopes of increasing the flow of their nervous fluid.

The development of portable machines to produce static electricity left the medical part of the field open to the showmen. Traveling entertainers put on shows that combined lectures about the new electricity with displays of static electricity that included the demonstration of sparks and the ability of static to literally make the hair stand on end.

The Medical Battery

The outcome of all this interest in electricity was a series of electrical devices, generically called an electric battery, which was a portable source for generating electricity. Today, this type of device would be referred to as an electrical generator, because of the method by which it generated electricity.

Electrical power is generated and supplied as two different types,

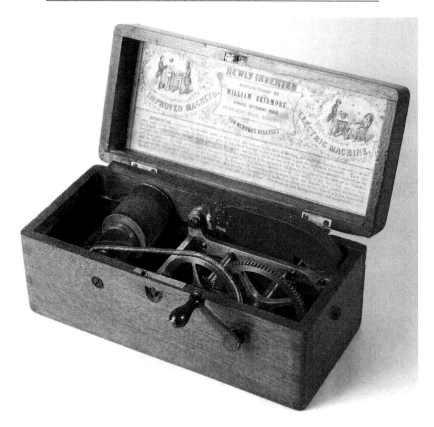

The Skidmore electrical generator was typical of the "medical batteries" that were designed to deliver an electrical current to the patient. When the handle at the front of the cabinet was turned, two coils inside the device rotated in front of a magnet and generated an electrical voltage that was delivered to the patient via two electrodes. This type of generator was commonly used for the treatment of "nervous diseases" (author's collection).

direct current (DC) and alternating current (AC). Direct current flows in only one direction, from the positive terminal of a battery through some type of circuit (in this case the patient) to the negative terminal.[16] Examples of direct current are the voltage produced by the cells used in flashlights and the batteries in automobiles. A single flashlight cell produces 1.5 volts and an automobile battery 12 volts.

Alternating current, as its name implies, alternates as it flows through the circuit, one terminal becoming positive and producing current flow to the other, then reversing (alternating) and becoming the negative terminal and receiving the current flow.[17]

The name "battery" is and has been used somewhat loosely, so it is important to clarify the meaning of the term. In technical terms, a device that converts chemical energy into an electrical energy source capable of providing an electrical current, such as a penlight flashlight battery, is correctly called a "cell." A series of cells wired together, such as the six lead-acid cells that make up a car battery, is called a "battery." This terminology, however, is not particularly important in everyday life and the name battery is generically applied to both.

The name "medical battery" in Victorian terms is further confusing as the name did not refer to a battery such as a flashlight battery, as the term is now known, but it was the name for the entire generating apparatus that provided direct current (which was referred to as "galvanic" current) or alternating current (often referred to as "faradic" current), or a combination of both. For galvanofaradization, also known as Watteville current, both galvanic and faradic currents were applied at the same time.

The medical battery was usually housed in a wooden box or cabinet. Even though most medical batteries provided both direct and alternating current, they were sometimes referred to as "faradic batteries." Various different methods were used to interrupt and pulse the direct current, thus producing a source of alternating current when desired.

To add to the confusion of battery terminology, wet-cell chemical batteries were also used to generate electricity. To use the Nonpareil chemical battery in 1855 the user had the messy task of mixing sulfuric acid and potassium bichromate in the cell to create the electrical voltage. Similarly, the early wearable electric belts generated a voltage by combining zinc and copper plates, separated by paper and soaked in vinegar. By the 1880s most equipment ran from dry-cell batteries, like those today, with the chemicals sealed inside a leak-proof housing.

A large number of electrical devices that claimed to cure a wide variety of ailments were developed by both legitimate and dubious inventors. Beginning in the mid–1800s, a medical battery was considered an essential part of every well-equipped physician's office equipment. These batteries were popular and in wide use between about 1870 and 1920. Many could be purchased directly by the patient and used in the privacy of their own home. Electricity was a new technology, but it was also perceived as mystical as it could not be seen or heard.

Electricity, however, could certainly be felt, and receiving an electrical tingle or shock made the patient feel like some sort of important treatment was taking place.

Treatments for various conditions used both direct current and alternating current electricity as each was intended to produce particular results. Most early electrical treatments used galvanic or direct-current electricity, so the term galvanic treatments came to have the same meaning as "medical electricity." One of the first machines was Davis & Kidder's Patent Magneto-Electric Machine, advertised as a cure for "nervous diseases."[18] The user applied two electrodes to the desired part of the body then cranked the handle of a generator which rotated an armature inside a magnet to deliver the electric current, similar to the way electricity is produced today by electrical generators.

A similar device was made by William Skidmore , a surgical instrument maker of Sheffield, England. His Improved Magneto-Electrical Machine was particularly recommended for the treatment of nervous diseases. It was also claimed to be useful for toothache, the facial pain of tic douloureux, and neuralgia. The faster the crank was turned, the higher the current, so that in this way the user could regulate the electric dosage.

Morehead's Graduated Magnetic Machine, first manufactured in 1847 in New York City, combined galvanic technology with mesmerist principles. Morehead sold his machine for twenty years through the mail. His machine, intended for home use, was essentially the same as the medical batteries sold to physicians. The device incorporated two metallic handles that were held by the user while the machine delivered current. The patients were supposed to feel a definite tingle in the hands and wrists.

Morehead claimed that disease was the result of "imperfect vital forces," and his machine was supposed to cure sickness by recharging the body with electricity that transferred energy and temporarily powered the body. Morehead had neither medical credentials nor extensive electrical knowledge, but was a tinkerer. He stated that his machine would revolutionize medicine, but never said how. He actually admitted that he would leave an understanding of how electricity worked to someone else, but did state that galvanism or magnetism was identical to vitality.[19]

To perform treatments with a medical battery, two electrodes were connected to the patient, with the current flowing between the two. One electrode was connected to one terminal of the source of electricity and the second electrode to the other. The patient's body then completed the electrical circuit back to the machine. A typical treatment involved the patient holding a cylindrical metal electrode in each hand as current was applied through the body. Current was generally applied for ten to twenty minutes in each session.

Some electrodes were made in the form of a flat metal plate that was placed against the body to conduct current into or out of it. Some of the plates were so large that the patient sat or stood on them. Smaller-sized plates were applied to specific parts of the body, such as the back or abdomen. Another form of electrode was a metal cylinder that was held in the hand. An electrode might also simply be a moistened cloth, perhaps soaked in saline solution to create better flow of current.[20]

Depending on the treatment, another method was to place a flat electrode in fixed contact with the body and then move the other electrode, in the form of a metal probe, over the skin around the abdomen, back, and neck. Some treatments were percutaneous, or external current applied through the skin, where both electrodes were placed in contact with the outside surface of the body. Others involved inserting one of the electrodes into a body cavity. Most medical batteries were supplied with a variety of different attachments, such as an eye-cup electrode for eye treatments, and electrodes for insertion into the natural body cavities (nose, ears, mouth, throat, vagina, and rectum) to provide other specialized treatments.

General faradization was used to treat the body as a whole and was recommended as a treatment when an illness was systemic in nature. For general faradization, one of the electrodes was placed underneath the patient's feet, sometimes with both the patient's feet and the electrode submerged in water to make better electrical contact, while the second electrode was moved over the head, spine abdomen, and other parts of the body, either by the patient or the physician. The current was applied for twenty to thirty minutes. By contrast, local faradization treated only a small part of the body and was used when a pain or illness was situated in a particular part of the body.

One legitimate, but unpleasant-sounding and highly-painful use for the rectal probe was for the treatment of hemorrhoids in a procedure called "anal faradism." The rectal electrode was inserted and a large jolt of electrical discharge was used to literally burn and cauterize the dilated veins in the hemorrhoids.[21]

Conventional physicians started to refer to electricity as the "life force itself," a description that was unfortunately quickly adopted by the quacks. By the 1880s numerous physicians were using electricity to treat patients, but at the same time quack medical practitioners expanded the use of electrotherapy to treat a wide variety of other ailments from poor eyesight to sexual problems, none of which were curable by electricity.

While the medical battery was developed for use in physicians' offices and was considered to be a legitimate treatment device for use by medical professionals, what were essentially the same devices quickly entered the consumer market. Medical textbooks and journals did not describe or encourage using medical electricity at home, but at the same time electrotherapy instrument manufacturers sold what they called "family batteries" for consumers to use on themselves in their own homes. As such, the machines occupied a difficult position in the medical world. They were considered to be devices used by professionals to provide legitimate therapy, yet at the same time they were promoted for home use. Some physicians were opposed to the use of electricity by uneducated consumers, in part because they felt it weakened the field of electrotherapy as a medical procedure. At the same time, other physicians were recommending the home use of medical electricity to their patients.[22]

Electric batteries for home use were mostly sold directly to consumers via newspaper advertisements and mail order marketing, and could be found in the catalogs of the major mail order companies, such as Sears, Roebuck between 1900 and 1920. In 1918 Sears offered three kinds of medical batteries costing from $4.95 to $11.95, three violet ray devices, and six models of vibrator, costing from $5.95 to a "professional" model for $28.95.[23]

Shocking Therapy

As early as 1869, W.R. Wells claimed in his book *A New Theory of Disease* that disease was an imbalance of the electrical forces in the body and that by applying electricity a practitioner could restore the balance and equilibrium.[24] Electricity was applied as galvanic, interrupted galvanic, faradic, galvanofaradic, sinusoidal, static, pulsed, static induction (Morton), or high frequency current. Pulsed current might use fast or slow alternations.

Direct or galvanic current produced stimulation of the skin and increased local circulation to produce absorption of inflammatory products. The electricity was applied to improve circulation to reduce swelling and overcome muscle spasms. Galvanic current was used to produce mild heat in cases of chronic or acute inflammatory conditions and circulatory disturbances.[25]

Another use for electric treatment was to give mild electric shocks in the hopes of restoring brain power. The theory was that energy would be transferred from the generating device to the body, though obviously electricity could not re-build damaged nerve endings or damaged tissue.

Faradic current, today called tetanizing current, was applied to muscles to give a continuous contraction during its entire flow. Galvanic current did not cause muscle contractions while flowing, but caused a brisk single contraction, a twitch, when suddenly started or stopped.[26] By the 1870s electrical treatments were mostly standardized, with physicians primarily using galvanic current.

The years from 1880 to 1920 were the golden age of electrotherapy, when electrical treatments were all the fashion, both by conventional physicians and manufacturers of quack medical devices. Physicians increasingly purchased and used medical batteries for office treatments. At the same time, the electrification of America reinforced the public's belief in electricity as the electric light spread across nation, followed by the telephone and the electric streetcar. As individual homes became connected to the electrical grid that was spreading across the country, newly-invented household electrical appliances, such as washing machines, toasters, sewing machines, teakettles, vacuum cleaners, and electric stoves, started to appear in private homes. And so did electrical treatment machines.

In 1873 Drescher's sold seventeen different electrotherapy machines at prices ranging from $10 to $250. In 1882, companies such as Jerome Kidder were offering electrical machines for use by physicians. Galvanic or faradic machines cost from $10 to $18, with a basic galvanic-faradic combination model costing $25. In 1888 Professor W.R. Wells offered a medical battery for home use, similar to that sold by Jerome Kidder, along with instructions for device maintenance and how to increase the machine's power.

By the 1880s electricity was applied to any body part that hurt. At the peak of the trend in the 1880s and 1890s, practitioners treated just about everything with electricity, especially neurasthenia and gyneco-logical problems. Patients had sessions in the "galvanic bath" and with the "magnetic machine." Textbooks of electrotherapy were common by 1900 and many hospitals had their own electrotherapy departments.

Electricity also offered hope that the trend of declining vitality with age could be reversed and the vigor of youth restored. Inventor Thomas Edison experimented with electricity for healing and developed the "inductorium" to cure rheumatism through electricity in a treatment where the user received electric shocks from an induction-coil device.[27] Edison's son, Thomas A. Edison, Jr., promoted a more questionable pseudo-medical device. He designed the Magno-Electric Vitalizer in the early 1900s and promoted it as an energy-enhancing device. His company was shut down for fraud in 1904 and he was arrested.[28]

The sale of electrotherapy equipment and electrical devices for the home was one of the most profitable categories of the proprietary health device business at the turn of the century.[29] However, as early as the late 1880s electrotherapeutic devices were starting to be viewed as question-able, even while they were still being widely advertised and sold. Con-fusion was generated in consumers' minds because legitimate medical doctors endorsed electrotherapy for legitimate medical uses. Thus it was an easy step for the charlatans to step in and offer electric cures for any-thing and everything. Because legitimate physicians used and endorsed electric devices, the public equally believed the charlatan. Anyone could administer treatments and medical batteries could be purchased by mail order for treating oneself at home. Thus, when considering the widespread use of treatment with electrical machines, the distinction between regular and unconventional medicine became blurred, and the promotion of the use of electricity for treatment by legitimate licensed physicians led to an unintended support of quacks and their suspect treatments. John Girdner quoted a specialist in *Munsey's* magazine in

April 1903 who said, "there are so many quacks and charlatans who deceive and rob the public by promises to cure disease with one electrical device or another that the medical profession is disposed to look askance at all such claims."[30]

Another problem for the conventional medical establishment was that physicians could not directly say that questionable electrical devices, such as electric belts, did not work, because many legitimate physicians and scientists of the time were also conducting their own research and experiments with electricity to determine the effectiveness of various treatments. Both doctors and patients usually relied on information supplied by the medical battery companies as they didn't understand electricity. The promise was that the internal electric force would recharge you for better health. The accompanying tingle meant that treatment was working.

Electrical Baths for Health

A common electrical treatment was the electric bath, also known as the "electrothermal bath," "electrohydric bath," or "electrogalvanic bath," intended to treat "nervous debility or exhaustion" in businessmen. The patient sat or reclined in a bathtub while small amounts of faradic, galvanic, or galvanofaradic electrical current were passed through the water and the patient.

The electric bath treatment became popular after the American Civil War, both as a medical treatment and a quack cure. The treatment was still in common use in the 1870s, essentially unchanged from the 1850s. The treatment used electrodes in a bathtub filled with warm water to apply electricity to the entire surface of the body. One of the electrodes for applying the current consisted of a series of metal plates mounted on the inside of a wooden or porcelain bathtub filled with water. The patient held the other electrode in his hand, submerged under the water, while a weak electrical current was passed between the two electrodes. In a similar type of arrangement, the patient rested his or her feet under the water near a large conductive electrode made from copper, lead, or carbon. The treatment was promoted for nervous and spinal afflictions, and neuralgia. For treatment with another type of electric bath, known as the Schnee Bath, the patient sat with his hands and feet in containers of water while an electric current was passed through them to the body.

In one type of electric bath, the patient reclined in the bathtub with only his head exposed. Gant explained the procedure: "After the tub had been filled and the patient has assumed the recumbent posture, the current is gradually turned on until a feeling of discomfort is complained of." This treatment with faradic, galvanic or galvanofaradic current lasted for fifteen to twenty minutes, then the patient was sprayed down with a cold jet of water.[31]

In the 1870s galvanic baths were used to treat impotence. George Schweig, a physician in New York, was well-known for his use of this type of treatment, which lasted for several minutes and was given up to six times a week. By the 1880s numerous physicians used electricity for similar treatments. George Beard and Alphonso Rockwell, the promoters of neurasthenia treatments, used a combination of localized galvanic current applied to the genitals and general galvanization with the current applied to the entire body.[32]

Another type of early electrical baths was the electrochemical bath, employed for the supposed removal of heavy metals from the body. Promoters of these electrochemical baths claimed that toxic metals, such as lead, mercury, and gold, that had been absorbed by workers as an occupational hazard of many industrial processes, could be removed from a patient by passing an electric current through the body to draw out the poisonous compounds.[33] Ironically, many of the heavy metals had actually come from the medical profession itself, which inadvertently poisoned patients with toxic heavy metals as part of drug treatments, such as the mercury in calomel, Fowler's Solution that contained arsenic, and purgatives containing antimony. People were quite willing to try a simple bath treatment that offered to remove the toxic metals that remained in their systems.

Promoters of the electrochemical bath built their advertising campaigns around the recently-developed principles of electrolysis, which was a legitimate industrial process used for plating objects by chemically moving conductive metals from one electrode to another with the use of electricity. By 1860, both Trall's Hydropathic and Hygienic Institute in New York and T.T. Seelye's Cleveland Water Cure Establishment offered electrochemical baths that were specifically advertised to extract metallic poisons from the body. This was another example of taking a scientific fact, in this case from electrochemistry and the use of electrolysis, combining it with a little wishful thinking, and coming up with a dubious treatment based on dubious science.

Electric Rings, Corsets and Brushes

While the medical battery emerged as a reputable medical treatment device, a variety of other "electrical" devices of a more questionable nature made their way onto the consumer market. In the late 1800s both popular magazines and learned periodicals were full of advertisements for "electric devices" with which to cure most of the ailments known to man. Typical were the electropathic belts, which claimed to cure diseases such as rheumatism, lumbago, sciatica, kidney complaints, paralysis, indigestion, gout, and a whole host of other diseases.

The Sears, Roebuck catalog offered a variety of "electric" medical devices for direct sale to the patient, including electric liniment, electric belts, magnetic insoles (at eighteen cents a pair), electric battery plasters, and electric rings. Many of the illustrations in the advertisements included little flashes of lightning shown coming from the devices. The 1880s saw advertisements for various electric garments to cure "nervous debility." Various types of electric clothing were popular, including electric belts, vests, socks, hats, garters, corsets, towels, and shoes. Many of these devices were advertised as being electric, galvanic, or magnetic.

Scott's Electric Corsets incorporated magnetized strips of metal which provided a "health giving current to the whole system." As a marketing gimmick each corset was supplied with a small compass so that the user could test and observe the magnetic power swirling through

Opposite: **Electric belts, which generated a voltage by combining zinc and copper plates separated by paper and soaked in vinegar, supposedly radiated electrical energy into the body. They were claimed to be effective for treating such diverse ailments as kidney disease, aching muscles, and deafness. First appearing on the market in the 1870s, these belts were worn around the waist for eight to twelve hours a day to allegedly remove the causes of disease and invigorate the nerves. Electric belts were the most popular impotence "cure" between 1890 and 1920, allowing men to do something in secret about any perceived sexual failings (author's collection).**

the garment for herself.[34] As well as the magnetic versions of corsets, some were electric and incorporated small batteries.

Harness' Electropathic (battery) Belt, sold by the Medical Battery

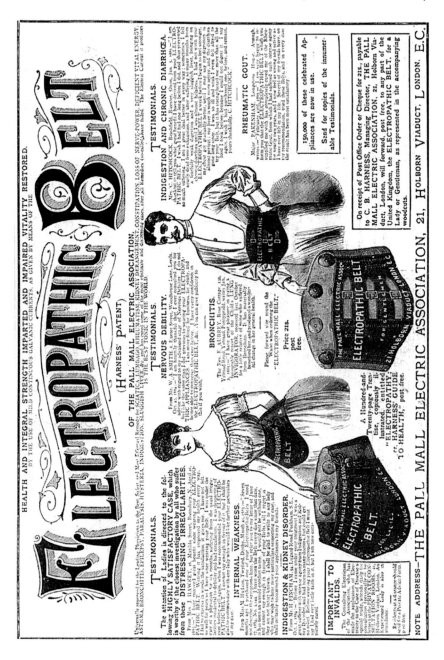

Company of London, was designed by C. Bennett Harness, listed in advertising as "The Eminent Consulting Medical Electrician" retained by the company for consultations. According to their advertising, "over a quarter of a million patients have been successfully treated for rheumatism, lumbago, sciatica, gout, kidney complaints, epilepsy, paralysis, indigestion, constipation, female complaints, general and local debility, functional disorders, etc."[35] In other words, almost every minor ailment that plagued most people was said to be treated.

Electric rings were popular among consumers. These rings were supposedly constructed from two different metals that would generate an electrical current when exposed to moisture or sweat from the body. They were supposed to cure anything and everything, though primarily aches and pains. The rings were to be worn on the third finger of the left hand, the same as a wedding ring. And for the same reason, because according to tradition there was a nerve or vein that led from that finger directly to the heart. For married customers, the electric ring could be worn next to the wedding ring.[36]

The Electro-Chemical Ring was developed by W.G. Brownson at the Electro-Chemical Ring Company of Toledo, Ohio. Brownson called himself a "medical electrician." His invention was an iron ring that retailed for $2. When worn on the finger, the ring was guaranteed to cure twenty-one different ailments, including diabetes, cancer, psoriasis, and epilepsy. Investigators did not agree, though the company managed to last for twenty-three years until it was finally shut down by the Post Office in 1914.[37]

Electripatent socks and insoles were claimed to prevent a leakage and loss of vital bodily electricity through the feet.[38] Another design of electric shoe insoles was sold as a pair, with one being copper and the other zinc. Supposedly the two different metals in contact with the body generated electricity as a type of battery. Current supposedly ran from one insole, up one leg and down the other to the other insole, infusing the body with electricity as it went.[39]

In 1916 a patent was issued to Dr. Frederick C. Werner for a Galvano Necklace, which was advertised by Cosmas Pharmacal Company as "the latest discovery for the relief of goiter [an enlargement of the thyroid gland] by mild electric treatment."[40] The necklace consisted of a series of pairs of zinc and copper plates, the plates of each pair separated by an insulator to create a series of small batteries. When in contact with moisture or sweat on the skin, the necklace was supposed to generate an electrical voltage. Reportedly it did not have much success.[41]

The Riley Electric Company of New Jersey produced an electric hairbrush in the 1890s that incorporated a small battery in the handle that supposedly applied electrical current to the hair. A similar device was the d'Argence Electric Brush. The brush contained a battery inside the hollow wooden housing of the handle. Like many of the other electric "brushes" it was recommended for curing baldness. The housing also contained two small electrodes for body use.

Dr. Scott's Electric Hairbrush, made by Dr. George Scott, looked like an ordinary hairbrush, but had a small magnetic rod embedded in the handle of the device. Scott had a clever sales gimmick. Each brush was supplied with a small compass. When the compass was placed near the brush, the compass needle moved, thus demonstrating to the consumer the mysterious electrical power that was contained in the brush.[42] As further testimony to the power of the brush, part of the carving on the back of the brush showed a muscular arm gripping a collection of four lightning bolts. One advertisement for Dr. Scott's Electric Hairbrush said that it was "Warranted to cure nervous headache in 5 minutes."[43] The back of the brush was adorned with carving that looked similar to a British royal seal, and the words "The Germ of All Life Is Electricity" around the outside. Dr. Scott's Electric Flesh Brush looked very similar, but had no handle.

The only power provided by these brushes was due to their internal magnets, therefore the "electric" brush was technically magnetic, but Scott preferred to advertise the brush as being electric. Among other ailments, the brush was intended to treat rheumatism, malaria, constipation, and diseases of the blood. Scott was versatile. In the 1880s he also sold magnetic belts and corsets, electric insoles, throat protectors, and leg appliances.

Scott was a clever marketer. He obtained several patents for his brushes; however, the patents were for the designs of the brushes, rather than their curative powers, which were never mentioned. Thus he was able to claim that the brushes were patented, inferring that their mode of curative action was so special that they were protected by a patent.

The Wonder Electric Generator, a small brush distributed exclusively by McKinley, Stone & Mackenzie of New York in 1922, was advertised to brush away the pain of headaches and rheumatism, as well as curing neuritis and the common cold. Serving double duty, it could be used on the face to improve the complexion. And, of course, like every other similar quack device, the brush could be used to relieve constipation by merely brushing the abdomen. The brush contained no batteries, but was powered by a tiny electrical generator inside the back of the brush that was activated by moving the thumb while brushing.[44]

Odds and Ends

Several cures for deafness used electricity. People suffering from deafness were advised to use Dr. Branaman's Combination Treatment, which involved treatment with an electromagnetic head cap while taking a series of proprietary medicines. The head cap consisted of a series of straps and metal pieces worn on the head that was supposed to send an electric current through the ears and thus re-vitalize damaged auditory nerves. It was powered by a battery pack in the head cap that had to be soaked in vinegar before use to activate the current flow. This miraculous head cap was only available from Dr. Branaman for a modest $8. Sales letters contained statements of this type: "Deafness cured in your own home" and "Stone deaf ... have heard whispers after my treatment."[45] The company was finally found guilty of postal fraud and was shut down.

A similar device was sold by Dr. Guy Clifford Powell from Peoria, Illinois, around 1905. The name was the Electro-Vibratory Apparatus for the Cure of Deafness. The machine supposedly cured deafness by pumping air in and out of the ears, at the same time sending shocks through the head that were applied via water-soaked electrodes inserted into the patient's ear canals.

Another odd device that was claimed to cure deafness was Wilson's Common Sense Eardrums, sold in 1892 by Wilson's Eardrums Company of Louisville, Kentucky. This was a kit that consisted of a tuning fork, a probe for cleaning wax from the ears, and a packet of boric acid powder to make a solution to rinse out the ear canals. The instructions explained how to use the probe and cotton wool soaked in boric acid to clean out the ears. In the sense that an ear canal completely blocked with earwax would indeed reduce hearing ability, cleaning out the wax would appear to the patient to restore hearing and cure deafness. The tuning fork could be used to test the newly-restored hearing ability.

The Electreat was a device promoted in the 1920s and 1930s to relieve pain. The mechanism consisted of flashlight batteries, a small electrical coil, and a door buzzer, along with attachments for application to various parts of the body. The device was essentially a hand-held roller and massager that created a series of electrical shocks that could be varied from a slight tingle up to 1,250 volts, that were supposed to relieve pain. The alleged concept was that forcing electricity into an area of the body forced the pain out. The accompanying instruction manual contained the frightening sentence that "pain is the messenger of death," and that electrical massage was the only way to relive it. The device allegedly "flushes out the sewers of our bodies" by increasing blood circulation. Among its many other recommended applications, such as to hands, back, neck, legs, and abdomen, the Electreat could be used on the scalp with a brush-like attachment for dandruff and falling hair, and to promote brain stimulation and restfulness. It was also claimed to treat deafness. The cost was only $15.[46] Needless to say, it was quickly seized by the FDA.[47]

Dr. Fred Urbuteit, a naturopath from Tampa, Florida, developed what he called a Sinuothermic Machine. The machine delivered a mild electrical current to the body to allegedly aid in the diagnosis and cure of various diseases and physical disorders such as cancer, diabetes, tuberculosis, arthritis, and paralysis. Various models of the machine were available from $1,500 to $3,000.[48] The devices were eventually seized and condemned.

SEVEN

Messing with the Mind

O ne of the prime targets for electrical treatments was a set of curious psychological illnesses that were a product of the Victorian age. One was a mental disease called neurasthenia that was thought to be brought on by the stresses of contemporary modern life, and showed up primarily in Victorian men in the second half of the nineteenth century. The corresponding mental disease found in women was hysteria, the primary symptoms of which would now be considered to be a combination of paranoia and manic depression.

Neurasthenia

In 1869 George Miller Beard, a pioneer in psychotherapy and a specialist in electrotherapy, first used the term "neurasthenia" to describe a set of mysterious ailments that was appearing primarily in urban middle-class white American men at mid-century. It was a peculiar condition of nervous exhaustion that appeared to be common in the northeast United States.[1] This vague mental disease did not appear to affect rural working men, such as farmers or common laborers, but was diagnosed only in the urban business class of workers where men had occupations that required them to use mental effort. Beard felt that this nervous exhaustion was a byproduct of society changing from a rural sedentary life to one of urban social, political, and economic struggle.[2] He noted that geographic areas of advanced industrialization in England and Germany also had high incidences of the disease.

Further study of this "nervous exhaustion," "brain exhaustion," and "spinal exhaustion" seemed to confirm Beard's original idea that neurasthenia was a weakness of white-collar workers. Beard eventually wrote half-a-dozen books on the subject.

Beard theorized that the amount of energy in the human body was finite and that the reserves of energy in the body were continually diminishing in strength. He argued that every individual was born with a fixed amount of energy to live their daily life and that once the energy was used up, there was no more. His explanation was that simple laborers were born with enough energy to complete all their tasks during their lifetimes, but educated men who used their brains for work required larger amounts of energy and used their energy up at a faster rate. Therefore, because modern urban life required increased amounts of energy, the city dweller was continually exhausted. The added result was the onset of wasting diseases such as consumption (tuberculosis), fatigue, nervousness, impotence, and heart palpitations.[3]

Beard claimed that neurasthenia was linked to increased intellectual development in the Victorian American male, and he saw it as a sign of his mental superiority. Beard distinguished between "muscle workers," who labored with their bodies in rural settings and "brain workers," such as doctors, lawyers, and inventors.

The symptoms of neurasthenia were nebulous, varied, odd, and vague. Patients showed symptoms of various diseases, but without any organic cause. Among other symptoms that were confusing to both the sufferer and the diagnostician, neurasthenia was said to be characterized by an extreme sensitivity to weather changes, tenderness in the teeth, gums, and scalp, fidgetiness, palpitations, excessive sensitivity to being tickled, itching, hot flashes, sweating hands, dyspepsia, writer's cramp, chills, hot flashes, muscle spasms, and yawning. Some sufferers exhibited sleeplessness and anxiety; others showed weariness and despondency, and a distaste for certain foods. One of the odder symptoms was a fear of the stars. Headaches, neck pain, groin discomfort, and limb atrophy were commonly reported to physicians. Symptoms were usually accompanied by fatigue, weakness, irritability, and an inability to concentrate, as well as various aches and pains. These manifestations seemed to be unlimited and Beard devoted a full page-and-a-half of dense small print to a list of symptoms in his book *American Nervousness: Its Causes and Consequences* (1881). And even he said that the list was not complete.

Beard claimed that the "nerve force" that the body possessed in limited amounts was being depleted by typical daily urban activities, including education, exercise, and employment that required mental activity. He postulated that this precious energy was also wasted on what he felt were unproductive illicit activities, such as the use of strong drink, gambling, involuntary nocturnal emissions, and masturbation, which were not surprisingly four of the activities high on the list of condemned items opposed by contemporary Victorian moralists and purity writers.

Men were obsessed with the fears of losing their manhood as a result of nocturnal emissions and masturbation, and frantically sought cures when they were diagnosed with neurasthenia.[4] Beard believed that any man suffering from neurasthenia was suffering also from sexual dysfunction and routinely questioned new patients in detail about the functioning of their genito-urinary system, which he believed was a frequent cause or contributor to the problem.

The body's vital energy was theorized to travel through the nerves and produce productive force. According to Beard, excessive thinking, mental work, physical activity, or sexual activity used far more energy than could be completely recovered during a normal period of rest. He claimed that the body required almost five times as long as the original activity to recover from any loss. Thus, the result was neurasthenia.

The loss of vital energy that was theorized to characterize neurasthenia had seemingly been confirmed in 1852 when William Thompson (Lord Kelvin), offered proof for the Second Law of Thermodynamics, which in one form basically said that energy was always being lost as it was converted from one form to another, and could never be restored to its original amount. Simply put, energy was in a constant state of decline. For example heat energy, such as that produced by a boiler, could be converted to mechanical energy, but during the process some of the energy was lost and could never be recovered. Applied to the human body, the more energy, particularly brain energy, that was used up due to the demands of civilization, the faster the person's individual supply ran down and was exhausted. The second part of the thinking was that the loss of vital bodily energy leading to neurasthenia could be replaced by infusing the body with external replacement energy, such as by giving the patient electric shocks or utilizing the energy provided by radium.

Neurasthenia and "nervousness" became a self-fulfilling medical prophecy. By the 1890s neurasthenia was accepted as a legitimate disease by the American medical community and became a frequent diagnosis for a wide variety of nebulous symptoms that seemed to be unlimited. Neurasthenia quickly became the predominant malady of late nineteenth-century culture. It supposedly accompanied the increased activities of civilized man that used steam power, the rotary press, the telegraph, and the other achievements of science. Beard even blamed an increase in nervous disease on the invention of the electric light.

Beard never really explained neurasthenia, and his claim that the nervous system went through "morbid changes in its chemical structure" was never verified by physiologists.[5] Beard considered neurasthenia to be a "state of disease," rather than a specific disease, though his interpretation of this fine distinction remained unclear and unexplained.

Hysteria

Hysteria was another imprecise diagnosis that was used to describe a similar series of nebulous symptoms in women. The affliction of hysteria appeared in Egyptian medical literature as early as 2,000 BC. The name of this ethereal disorder was derived from *hystera*, the Greek name for the uterus.

One description of hysteria was that it "…is characterized by a grumbling noise in the bowels; a sense of suffocation as though a ball was ascending to the throat; stupor, insensibility, convulsions, laughing and crying without any visible cause; sleep interrupted by sighing and groaning, attended with flatulence and nervous symptoms. It is caused by affections of the womb, &c."[6]

Like neurasthenia, hysteria was accompanied by various nervous and mental symptoms that could be related to almost every type of physical disease. Among other vague symptoms of the disease were headaches, fainting, insomnia, depression, morbid and unfounded fears, laughing and crying for no reason, nervousness, odd sensations in the abdomen, shortness of breath, muscle spasms, loss of appetite, amnesia, tremors, vomiting, sleep-walking, limb paralysis, and psychotic episodes.

The manifestation of symptoms was considered to be composed of three related disorders: hysteria, chlorosis, and neurasthenia. The symptoms of all three (as they were then defined) were similar and overlapping. The term "chlorosis," often used interchangeably at the time with hysteria, was a disease of young women that was also thought to have a uterine origin. It was alternately called "greensickness," because the victim's complexion took on a greenish hue. At the time, the cause was variously attributed to anemia, anorexia, or hysteria.

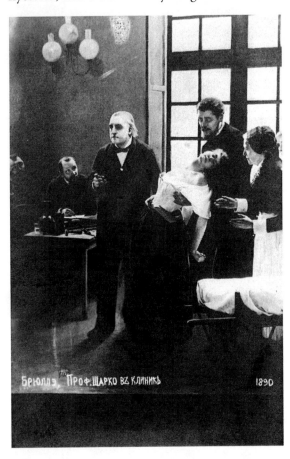

Greek physicians blamed hysteria on the uterus, which they felt became inflamed, or somehow became detached and moved around through the body. By the nineteenth century, physicians of course realized that the uterus was permanently attached in place by muscles and ligaments, but still continued to blame it for vague mental disorders of women. In view of this "enlightened" thinking, hysteria was theorized to

Hysteria was a mysterious yet common diagnosis in the late 1800s and early 1900s. This black-and-white postcard from 1890 features French neurologist and professor of pathology Jean-Martin Charcot, who expanded on the work of Franz Mesmer in hypnotizing subjects. Here Charcot is demonstrating the use of hypnosis on a hysterical female patient. The woman appears to have fainted and is being supported by an assisting doctor (National Library of Medicine).

be due to factors such as bad physical or moral education, living in a city, overindulgence in coffee and tea, and a bad constitution. Hysteria encompassed a wide set of symptoms that varied greatly between individuals and, like neurasthenia, functioned as a catch-all category for various undiagnosed conditions.

After 1900, the diagnosis of neurasthenia was also applied to women, making hysteria, chlorosis, and neurasthenia three interchangeable and confusing nebulous diseases. Physicians agreed that sufferers were typically men from stressful white-collar jobs, such as businessmen, salesmen, managers, writers, lawyers, and the other professions, but also women who were overly stressed by the incompatibility between intellectual pursuits and their roles as wives and mothers.[7] Reference sources on all three diseases are confusing and often contradictory, and the meanings of the terms have changed over time.[8]

Treating Neurasthenia

By the late 1800s scientists and physicians believed that the victims of neurasthenia were losing vital energy from the body faster than they could replace it. Physicians thought of the flow of nerve energy in the body in electrical terms, thinking of it as the flow of current in and out of a battery, like tides of electricity flowing in and out of the body. When these currents were disturbed, they thought the result was neurasthenia, hysteria, chlorosis, dyspepsia, and other supposedly severe conditions. They speculated that sources of external energy, such as electricity and later radioactivity, could recharge the human body, so treatments for neurasthenia were intended to stop the dissipation of vital energy, and furthermore to recharge and re-energize the system. Because of its supposed relationship to electricity, neurasthenia was commonly treated by the use of electrical gadgets, thus restoring the body's "conductibility" and settling down the "molecular perturbations."[9]

The cure for neurasthenia depended on the gender of the patient. Physician S. Weir Mitchell prescribed rest in bed for at least a month for women, with no reading to excite their minds, and a milk-heavy diet that was fed to them with a spoon by a nurse. Men were advised to seek plenty of fresh air and exercise.[10]

After the development of electrotherapy devices, the popular form of treatment for neurasthenia was electrical stimulation that used various electrodes applied either to the skin or inserted into various body openings. One device that was widely advertised to offer a cure was a form of electric hairbrush. A more specific treatment was central galvanization, where patients sat with their feet on a sheet of copper attached to the negative pole of a medical battery. The positive pole was connected to an electrode to apply electrical current around the patient's head, back, spine, arms, abdomen, and legs.

George Beard and his professional partner Alphonso D. Rockwell used static, galvanic, and faradic currents to treat neurasthenia and other nervous ailments. For Beard's general faradization treatments, current was applied to the entire body. One copper electrode was attached to the patient's feet and the other held in his hand while current was allowed to flow between the two for ten to twenty minutes to induce muscular contractions. This treatment was intended to restore healthy circulation by replenishing the supply of energy if it was diminished—or if present, to redistribute it to useful areas of the body. Beard and Rockwell published the primary textbook, *A Practical Treatise on the Medical and Surgical Uses of Electricity*, on the subject.

The vague symptoms that characterized neurasthenia were thought to frequently change as the disease moved around to various parts of the body, thus it was thought that what was actually nervous prostration could show up as a digestive problem or a reproductive disturbance. To include all these changing symptoms, neurasthenia was categorized into different types, such as cerebral, spinal, digestive, traumatic, hysterical, or sexual.

As a result, a flood of neurasthenic men and women went to socially-accepted health resorts in the United States and Europe for treatments where they were subjected to shocks from electric belts, electrodes inserted into the urethra, various bowel treatments, magnetism, galvanism, drugs, and medicinal baths. One of the odder treatments was the use of animal "extracts" to try to stimulate nerve-cell activity. The Goat Lymph Sanitarium Association used animal extracts in a brain and nerve tonic. One peculiar treatment was to add extracts from animal brains to the individual's diet. Another was to inject into the abdomen a solution of sheep brains that had been ground into a pulp.[11]

According to physicians, perhaps not surprisingly for the times, difficulties with the sex organs were frequently considered to be the origin of neurasthenia and nervous exhaustion, and a variety of medicines and treatments were often concentrated on the genitals. Beard used a combination of localized galvanic current applied directly to the genitals, while other practitioners used both faradic and galvanic current.

This therapeutic use of electricity by legitimate medical doctors seems appalling in today's terms. The application of static, dynamic, or interrupted current applied to the spine, perineum, testicles, and penis was obviously painful. There was some reported success, but even one doctor who promoted the treatments described the effect as "rather unpleasant."[12] In even stronger terms was this quote from S.H. Monell, a professor of static electricity and secretary of the American Medical Association, in *A System of Electrotherapeutics* (1902). He said, "[T]he faradic brush applied to the testicles … gives excellent results … twenty or thirty applications are required to effect a cure … 1 or 2 minutes on each side; the current should be … strong, so that a distinct burning sensation is produced."

In a more severe form of treatment, one of the electrodes was inserted into the rectum and the other into the urethra, and electrical current applied between the two. This method was also recommended as treatment for cases of gonorrhea. Alternately, one electrode was placed in the rectum and the other applied to the perineum, the area between the genitals and the anus, or the inner side of the thighs. In using this method, Beard said, "…very strong currents can be applied."[13]

Ultzmann showed that an erection could be achieved by applying either continuous or faradic current with one electrode in the rectum and the other on the bulb of the urethra, thus it is possible that part of the apparent willingness of men to undergo such treatments may have been due to induced unusual or pleasurable sensations, as ejaculation was observed to be a common side effect of rectally administered electrotherapy.[14]

Another general treatment was called Franklinization, which involved a discharge of static electricity that was applied to the spinal and genital regions. The patient was seated on an insulated chair while the physician applied "electric wind" to his body with a variety of electrodes attached to a static electricity generator. Franklinization was often accompanied by passing mild current between electrodes inserted in the urethra and rectum.[15]

Even odder than these treatments was the vibrating urethral sound, which consisted of a metal probe attached to a large coiled metal spring. After the probe was inserted into the urethra, the spring was struck with a padded mallet so that the resulting vibrations were transmitted up the device into the urinary system. This treatment was used in cases of "relaxation, over-stimulation, and sexual neurasthenia."[16]

In spite of all this, being diagnosed with neurasthenia was not considered to be all bad by some patients because it became a rationalization for the superiority of urban life, a belief in the greater brain power of the urban business class, and a justification of the superiority of urban culture over traditional rural values.

Neurasthenia remained a mystery. Even by the 1890s, neither Beard nor anyone else had been able to detect any physiological cause for neurasthenia or observe any physical changes in patients caused by the "disease."[17] By 1903 even Rockwell had to admit that he did not understand why treatment worked. He further said that researchers were wrong about the nature of electricity. He decided that electricity was not a fluid at all, and that there was no neural fluid. And in 1904 Beard admitted that he didn't have any idea of how electrotherapy worked on neurasthenia and could find no physiological evidence for its efficacy.[18]

No pathology related to neurasthenia was ever discovered and electrical treatments of neurasthenia gradually lost favor as electrical stimulation failed to work more often than not. The obsession with neurasthenia started to fade in the early 1900s and was gone as a diagnosis by the 1920s.

Professional support for electrotherapeutics also started to decline by 1900 as neurasthenia lost its status as a pathological diagnosis, and gynecological problems were treated more effectively by surgery. Electrical stimulation was, however, retained as a treatment for autointoxication, as will be discussed later. By 1920 the use of electricity was falling out of favor for all types of treatment.

Eventually, general medical agreement was that hysteria was probably caused by sexual deprivation, as it most often affected young unmarried women, nuns, and widows. In the eighteenth and nineteenth centuries, marriage and intercourse were the accepted recommendation for a cure. If this option was not available, physicians recommended manual stimulation by a midwife to bring on the "hysterical paroxysm," which had the same indications as orgasm. This sounds suspiciously similar to what happened to the patients of Franz Mesmer, who was widely suspected of stirring up sexual passions and subsequent convulsive fits in his female patients.[19]

Treatments for hysteria also consisted of various other unusual therapies, such as using high-pressure jets of hot and cold water to buffet the body, flogging the patient with wet towels or sheets, or the old standby of purging to rid the body of decaying waste products that might be accumulating in the lower abdomen around the sex organs.

EIGHT

Advanced
Electrical Quackery

The use of medical devices based on electricity blossomed, starting in about 1870 and going strong until about 1930. Americans suffering from various ailments, both mild and severe, eagerly pursued alternative electrical therapies, paying little attention to cautions from the medical profession. Quacks quickly realized that many potential customers wanted inexpensive, easy-to-use products that promised to relieve aches and pains, revitalizes nerves, rejuvenate tired muscles, and cure a variety of other ailments for use in privacy in their own homes.

At the same time that physicians were waging war on the use of unapproved electrical treatment machines, an eager public was purchasing all sorts of outlandish medical devices, such as electric belts, ozone generators, violet ray machines, vibration mechanisms, and magnetic coils, to improve their health. Among the most popular devices were electric "invigorators," such as electric belts and magnetic collars. These devices were promoted to "energize" the body by replacing lost nerve energy and creating new energy.

Some of the "electrical" devices were, of course, completely bogus and ineffective. For example, Nolan's Famous Catarrh Cure was advertised as being electric pills with 50,000 volts of electricity in them.[1] Similarly the Galvano Necklace, which was recommended for treating goiter (an enlarged thyroid), was tested by the Post Office in 1930 and found to produce no electrical current at all.[2]

Brewster's Medicated Electricity claimed to have "a perfect electric battery in every bottle." This elixir of vegetable compounds, indeed with a small battery in every container, was claimed to be "an infallible remedy for headache, neuralgia, hay fever, catarrh, and cold in the head." It was also promoted as being useful for failing eyesight and deafness.

The Electric Belt

One of the more peculiar, but very popular, electric treatments of the time involved the use of electric belts to supposedly radiate energy into the body. These belts, the first of which appeared on the market in the 1870s, were electrical devices worn around the waist for eight to twelve hours a day to allegedly remove the causes of disease and invigorate the nerves through the use of electric currents. These belts were supposedly effective for treating such diverse ailments as kidney disease, aching muscles, deafness, and morphine addiction.

Electric belts were first marketed in the United States in 1875 by British electrician Isaac Lewis Pulvermacher. His belt consisted of a leather and cloth support with 120 coils of copper wire woven into the inside. Where the copper contacted the skin, electrodes produced a mild tingling sensation as electrical current passed through the coils.[3] The belt was sold as cure for rheumatism, gout, indigestion, paralysis, stiff joints, deficiency of nervous energy, and all nervous disorders.[4]

Pulvermacher developed telegraph machines and telegraphing techniques before perfecting and producing his electric belts. But even before making electric belts, in 1855 Pulvermacher had developed and described a type of voltaic battery device named the Pulvermacher Hydro-electric Chain. This consisted of a series of interconnected wooden cylindrical rods, spirally-wrapped with copper and zinc wires in the form of a chain, that looked somewhat like a miniature rope bridge. An electrode wired to each end of the "chain" was placed in contact with the patient's body to perform the "electrification" treatment. The length of the chain (the number of battery cells) determined the output voltage. The chains that had 120 cells were reported to be "quite strong." The entire device was soaked in diluted vinegar before use to add an electrolyte to activate the electrical cells. The basic chain produced galvanic (direct) current. A clockwork-driven interrupter could be included in the circuit to produce faradic (pulsed) current.

The electric chain was later replaced by various designs of electric belts. Pulvermacher originally manufactured his electric belts in London, but moved from England to Cincinnati in the 1880s because he saw that greater profits could be made in the United States. His was a truly international company as his devices were sold in Great Britain, France, Germany, Austria, Belgium, Canada, and the United States. Pulvermacher belts cost $20 each.[5] The slogan for Pulvermacher's Galvanic Company was "Electricity Is Life," and his advertising sketches included prominent flashes of electricity coming from the belts. He claimed that electricity was "Nature's Chief Restorer."

Early versions of the Pulvermacher belt had to be soaked in a diluted vinegar solution (acetic acid, a weak acid; one part vinegar to three parts water) before each use to activate the action of the battery and produce current to power the device. Later versions contained small sealed batteries inside the belt.[6] Similarly, in 1915 the Lorenz Truss and Electric Works in Chicago incorporated a dry cell battery for powering their belts.

By 1900 the Pulvermacher belt had been joined on the market by the German Electric belt, Edison's belt (from inventor Thomas Edison's son, Thomas Edison, Jr.), Dr. Crystal's, Addison's Electric Belt, the A.P. Owens belt, Dr. Horn's belt, the Boston Electric Belt, and the Heidelberg Electric Belt. Similar were Dr. Bridgman's Belt, Dr. Bell's Electro Appliance, the Lorenz belt, and the Electra-Vita Body Battery.

In spite of their impressive European names, the German Electric Company was based in New York City and Pulvermacher's of London, although it was originally founded in London, was based in Cincinnati in the United States. Belt manufacturers often used European names, such as the Heidelberg Electric Belt, to make the belts appear as though they were the product of superior electrical science from Europe.

Most belts claimed to be successful in treating nearly everything. For example, the Medical Battery Company of London sold Harness' Electropathic Belt for 21 shillings.[7] Advertising for the Electropathic Belt claimed that their device would successfully treat epilepsy, shortness of breath, asthma, constipation, weakness, dyspepsia, piles (hemorrhoids), bad circulation, consumption, neuralgia, hysteria, female irregularities, paralysis, muscle pains, writer's cramp, spinal weakness, general internal weakness, rheumatic fever, sciatica, kidney disorders, gout, bronchitis, nervous headache, nervous exhaustion, nervous debility, rheumatism, indigestion, and liver complaints.[8]

Despite hyperbole in their marketing claims, all the electric belts on the market were basically similar in operation and action. They typically consisted of a series of zinc disks connected together with a copper wire, with the whole arrangement built into a supporting belt made of leather and cloth. The belts were soaked in a dilute vinegar solution before each use to create a crude battery that generated a weak electrical current that was delivered through electrodes in contact with the body. Some batteries used a salt solution instead of vinegar. The current created a temporary mild tingling sensation in the skin where the metal electrodes touched.

Some companies tried to distinguish themselves by their advertising claims. Advertising for Dr. C.N. West's Electro Medical Belt, patented in 1878, stated: "This belt ... produces a *peculiar* current such as no other battery in the world can produce, and which perfectly adapts it to the human body, producing in it the same activity in all its various organs that the *vital* or *nerve* force usually performs in health" [italics in the original]. In an effort to distinguish itself, the German Electric Suspensory belt claimed that it contained four batteries in order to provide additional power.

Advertising for the German Electric belt claimed that passing a current through the body removed the causes of disease and invigorated the nerves that controlled their action. In one advertisement, the German Electric Belt Company capitalized on the new invention of electric household power and compared the application of electricity to the body via its belt to the revolutionary changes made by the introduction of the electric light, the telephone, and the telegraph. In so many words, it welcomed the consumer to the awesome technology of tomorrow.

The German Electric Belt Company credited the inventor of their belt as P.H. Van der Weyde, M.D., president of the New York Electrical Society.[9] Manufacturers of questionable medical devices often used the names and credentials of renowned physicians and scientists to authenticate their devices and claims, though sometimes the testimonials and people were as bogus as the devices.

Electric belts were heavily promoted in local and national newspapers, and in popular national magazines, such as *Harper's Weekly* and

The Illustrated News. Advertising usually contained glowing testimonials from alleged users, mixed in with a smattering of pseudo-scientific language. In spite of such language, these rambling discourses usually never actually said how the belts worked. To the uneducated reader, however, all this verbiage seemed like a scientific explanation, and the belts obviously met a popular demand.

For those who wanted to treat themselves at home, electric belts were sold by mail order houses, appearing in catalogs such as those from Sears, Roebuck for as little as $4.[10] The 1900 Sears catalog offered readers the Giant Power Heidelberg Electric Belt for $18.[11] In this way, the belts could be purchased in private and delivered to the buyer's home by mail with the utmost discretion for imagined problems of sexual inadequacy and other problems that most men would not even want to share with their family physician.

Unfortunately, misinformation abounded in much of the advertising copy. One of the devices that Sears, Roebuck sold in their catalog was the Heidelberg Alternating Current Medical Electric Belts. This was incorrect as the belts used a chemical battery that produced only a weak amount of direct current. Further nonsense was contained in the advertising copy for the $4 version which said, "This belt produces a 20-gauge current of electricity…" recommended for "mild cases." This sentence is meaningless in technical terms as electrical current is measured in amperes, not in wire gauge size. The $6 version claimed, "This 30-gauge current belt is strong enough for all ordinary forms of disease and weakness…." Again a meaningless phrase from an engineering standpoint. In fact, wire sizes are inversely proportional to their gauge, so a 20-gauge wire actually is larger than and has far more current carrying capacity than a 30-gauge wire.[12]

Representations of lightning bolts were often incorporated into advertising for electric belts to dramatize the power of the products. The Pulvermacher Galvanic Company used this visual aid to hint that the power of lightning was harnessed in their belts. Another favorite piece of symbolism was to show representations of sparks coming out of the belt. Illustrations in 1890 for the Owens electric belt, made by the Owens Electric Belt and Appliance Company, incorporated tiny bolts of lighting coming from the belt and the places where its electrodes contacted the body.[13] The Heidelberg Electric Belt in the Sears, Roebuck catalog showed a gaudy apparatus with similar lightning bolts spraying out of it. In reality, showing sparks and lightning bolts had nothing to do with the operation of the belt and had no basis in fact, as the belts (one hopes) did not emit any sparks or lightning bolts during operation. The batteries created only a very low level of current that produced a mild tingling in the skin.

To promote an association in the consumer's mind between the power of electricity and the electric belts, the cover of a pamphlet for the German Electric Belt Agency, titled "The Electric Age," showed Miss Liberty holding one of the new electric lights that were still a wonder to many people, especially rural buyers.

Electric belts were also sold directly from the factory by aggressive door-to-door salesmen. Salesmen's expansive claims generally went beyond what regular physicians were willing to state. Door-to-door peddlers capitalized on the general public's fear of disease and their fantasies of the curative power of electricity. Outlandish claims were made for the efficacy of these belts, promising a wide range of cures and catering to many people's general fear of disease.

The sale of electric belts was very profitable. Most electric belts sold for 25¢ to $2, but a variety of models and sizes sold from $4 to $18. The basic version of Addison's Electric Belt sold to the consumer for $1.10, but the wholesale cost to the salesman was $2.50 a dozen, or about 21¢ each. The Electric Appliance Company, makers of Addison's Electric Belt, advertised in *Billboard* in 1910 that salesmen could make 500 percent to 1,000 percent profit when selling their belts.

Direct mail solicitation was also used. Electric belts were sold by mail order houses because, in this way, they could be purchased in private and delivered to the buyer's home with the utmost discretion. The price was whatever the sales force felt that the market would bear, and might decrease dramatically in successive sales letters, depending on how long it took for the customer to answer the series of solicitation letters and buy a belt. In 1890 the German Electric Belt Agency occasionally offered their $5 belt for as low as $2 to try to encourage reluctant customers.

The Pulvermacher Galvanic Company sold belts to both men and women, though the belts aimed at women looked more like a corset, to conform to contemporary gender roles. Though electric belts were sold to cure many disorders, most advertising aimed at men was focused towards treating problems of the male reproductive organs for men who wanted to enhance their "performance," "restore the vital spark," or "renew lost manhood" through the new wonder of electricity.

To restore male hopes, the Pulvermacher belt had an optional accessory called a "suspensory appliance." This consisted of a light-weight wire mesh and cloth pouch that fastened to the belt, enclosing the genitals, and applied a mild galvanic current to the penis and testicles. It was advertised to restore "lost vigor" and "decline," both of which were well-known contemporary code words for a loss of sexual potency. To verify their point, typical print advertising showed electric lightning flashes radiating from electric belts, particularly in the area of the scrotum.

Morehead's Graduated Magnetic Machines similarly encouraged prospective consumers to improve their "vitality of life." Addison's Galvanic Electric Belt with its copper and zinc battery was marketed as "Nature's Vitalizer." Dr. Dye's Voltaic Belt claimed to cure "nervous debility, lost vitality, and loss of nerve force and vigor."[14] They essentially offered to create a new man by powering his genitals with electricity. Between about 1850 and 1930, the discreet terms "vim," "vigor," "vitality," and "virility" were all used as euphemisms for sexual power. In an effort to provide some sort of credibility for the consumer, this was essentially the same language for impotence and erectile disorders that the medical community was using.

Use of the device was probably not harmful; in fact the motion picture *The Road to Wellville* (1994) shows William Lightbody (Matthew Broderick) rather enjoying wearing one. However, the associated problem was that sales by mail order encouraged self-treatment at home instead of going to a doctor in the event of a serious condition.

Some of the advertising showed how to place and wear the belt on the body, and was usually illustrated by idealized sketches of naked men with strong arms, muscular thighs, and well-shaped virile bodies wearing the device.[15] They were typically posed wearing only the belt with the attached genital pouch, with their muscles flexed and their arms raised in positions of action. In this manner, a man's overall physical power in the modern world was equated to powerful genital functioning. The objective was to create the impression in the reader that he too could increase his physical characteristics, erectile performance, and sexual prowess by purchasing and wearing an electric belt. The advertisement did not depict most men as they were, but as what they hoped to become by buying the product.

Belt manufacturers played up the fear of various male problems and emphasized gloomy symptoms of sexual inadequacy in order to induce the fear of sexual failure in potential customers and thus sell more belts. Though electric belts did not and could not cure most physiological ailments, this does not mean that they were unimportant. The psychological results for the user could be useful if they gave him more confidence. Use of these gadgets started to decline in the 1920s and most had fallen from popular favor by the 1940s.

The I-ON-A-CO

When the popularity of the battery-operated electric belts started to decline in the 1920s, they were replaced by newer electrical products intended to appeal to the consumer.

In 1925, there was a renewed interest in magnetic treatment when Gaylord Wilshire of Los Angeles marketed what he called the I-ON-A-CO. This was an electric coil, worn around the neck or waist, that supposedly healed by magnetizing iron in the blood and treating body cells with electricity. It was claimed to be a sure cure for heart disease, cancer, diabetes, and prostate problems. The unusual name I-ON-A-CO was simply a flagrantly abbreviated version of "I-OWN-A-COMPANY." The more popular common nickname was the "horse collar."

The I-ON-A-CO consisted of a large coil of insulated wire, covered with leather, that was energized by plugging it into an electrical outlet. The device was hung from the patient's neck or placed around the waist and used for a recommended treatment time of ten to fifteen minutes each day to supposedly magnetize iron in the patient's blood. The manufacturer claimed that it worked by charging the body with electromagnetic energy to speed up the circulation and cure disease. The company referred to the I-ON-A-CO as "a simple and effective method of using magnetism for the cure of human ailments."[16] One advertisement for the I-ON-A-CO said, "It magnetizes the iron in your body and thus increases oxygen brought to the tissue cells. This oxygen purifies the blood stream and tends to restore the Ionaco user to perfect health."

The I-ON-A-CO was the brainchild of Henry Gaylord Wilshire, a California business tycoon who had previously made a fortune in Los Angeles real estate. Among his other accomplishments, Wilshire Boulevard, which travels west from downtown Los Angeles to the Pacific Ocean at Santa Monica, was named after him. Wilshire started marketing the I-ON-A-CO in 1925, supposedly as a cure-all. Wilshire had no medical training and his product had no scientific merits, but he became the leading

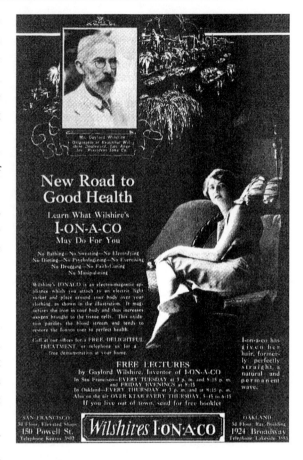

The I-ON-A-CO was a magnetic belt developed by Gaylord Wilshire in 1925. It was advertised to create a magnetic force around the body to stimulate the iron in the blood to greater action, thus increasing the body's absorption of healthy oxygen. Scientific fact was extrapolated into dubious theory to produce a device that nevertheless continued to sell well through the 1930s and 1940s (Wikimedia Commons).

producer of magnetic belts, selling thousands of them over a ten-year period.[17]

Wilshire based his concept for a magnetic belt on the fact that the body's red blood cells carried hemoglobin, which contained an iron ion bound inside it. Wilshire built on this small piece of science and, like many other questionable promoters, expanded on it and theorized (without any proof) that his belt would create a ring of magnetic force around the body to stimulate the iron in the blood to greater action, thus increasing the body's absorption of healthy oxygen. Without this energized field, he said that the body suffered from "auto toxemia" caused by poisons trapped in the tissues.[18]

Advertising for the I-ON-A-CO was an excellent example of starting with a small amount of legitimate science and then extrapolating it into blue-sky theory and bogus claims. A 1927 newspaper advertisement for the I-ON-A-CO said, "The I-ON-A-CO is based upon the recent discovery of Dr. Otto Warburg, the great German Biologist, that the iron in the system acts as a catalyzer or transfer agent uniting the oxygen we inhale with our tissue cells." The advertising copy here talked about the fact that hemoglobin in blood carried oxygen from the lungs through the bloodstream. This scientific fact was correct. But it was then extrapolated into dubious theory when it said that the I-ON-A-CO magnetized the blood, and "Through magnetization, the I-ON-A-CO improves the catalytic value of the iron—thus enabling it to deliver an increased supply of oxygen to the system." Furthermore, it claimed, "Wilshire's I-ON-A-CO is the first device ever discovered which improves this catalytic value."[19]

An example of the bogus testimonials used to promote the device was one from W.F. Brady, M.D., "Dean of the Faculty at the School of Electro Therapy at the University of Michigan." Upon investigation, it turned out that there was no School of Electro Therapy or any Dr. Brady at the university.[20]

Wilshire also incorporated a clever marketing gimmick, somewhat like Dr. Scott's use of a small compass to demonstrate the power of his magnetic hairbrush. A feature of the I-ON-A-CO that was intended to convince the consumer of the effectiveness of the power radiating from the device was a smaller secondary coil of insulated wire with the two ends attached to a small light bulb. When this smaller coil was brought close to the main coil after it was plugged-in, the light bulb lit up. Activation of the lamp without being plugged into any apparent power source was supposed to demonstrate the power and effectiveness of the I-ON-A-CO, as well as show the user that the device was working. In reality, this was simply a common electrical transformer principle that lit the bulb in the secondary coil through induction.[21]

When the I-ON-A-CO first went on the market, the sales price was $58.40 if purchased with cash or, if the customer chose the credit plan, with easy payments of $5 a month for a total cost of $65.[22]

The device was heavily promoted in newspapers and by door-to-door salesmen. They did their job so well that more than 3,000 of the devices were sold during the first year of business. The company prospered and opened Oregon in Portland, Eugene, Oregon City, and Roseburg as well as in Seattle and Tacoma. By 1927 the company had twenty-three regional offices. Approximately 50,000 belts were sold between 1925 and 1927.[23] The I-ON-A-CO continued to sell well through the 1930s and 1940s. The American Medical Association continued to refer to it as a "magnetic horse collar" and, after investigating the device, politely said that it was not good for curing anything. The Association repeatedly tried to tell the public that the belt had no merit, but sales continued to be brisk.[24]

Similar products that made up the competition were the Theronoid, Electronet, Magnecoil, Iona-tone, Restoro, and Master Circletone. In late 1926 the Portland Better Business Bureau investigated a device called the Mag-Kuro created by a pair of entrepreneurs named MacDonald, a businessman, and Johnson, an electrician, who planned to open a clinic in Tacoma.[25]

The Theronoid was a magnetic belt that was said to remove harmful waste products from the body while treating chronic ailments.[26] The Theronoid was almost the same as the I-ON-A-CO except that it had an on-off switch, which the I-ON-A-CO did not. The similarity was probably not surprising as the Theronoid was a direct descendant of the I-ON-A-CO. It was created in 1928 by Philip Isley, who had worked in Wilshire's Cleveland office.

In 1928 Magnecoil Company of Salt Lake City advertised that their device would cure by "promoting perfect elimination by cleaning the body inside and out." The recommended method of use was to place the Magnecoil on a couch and lie down on it as often as possible.[27]

The Electropoise and the Oxydonor

One of the early "electrical" devices heavily marketed to women was the Electropoise, a device that was advertised as inducing oxygen into the system via a metal plate fastened around the ankle, and was intended to combat the effects of fatigue and aging.

The inventor of the Electropoise was Dr. Hercules Sanche, who grandly called himself "The Discoverer of the Laws of Spontaneous Cure of Disease."[28] When Sanche first patented and marketed his oxygen device in 1892, he called it the Electropoise, a home remedy device that sold for $10 and reportedly allowed the human body to absorb additional oxygen for improving the healing process.

The Electropoise was a brass cylinder a little more than three inches long that weighed five ounces. The cylinder was closed at both ends and sealed. It had an attached flexible cord that came out of one of the ends. The other end of the cord was attached to a small metal plate that was fastened to the wrist or ankle via an elastic band and buckle. As Sanche explained the operation of the device, "The gases from decaying food are positive in their electrical quality and cause disease. With the Electropoise we cause the negative elements so abundant in the atmosphere to be attracted into the body in sufficient quantity to consume the accumulation of combustible matter stored up by the imperfect action of the vital organs." When the sealed cylinder was opened by scientists from the American Medical Association, the interior was found to be empty.[29]

Part of the popularity of the device may have been an appeal to sufferers of tuberculosis, which was rampant at the time. Advertisements for the Electropoise showed pale and thin women with fatigued expressions on their faces, which implied tuberculosis, even though this was not stated outright.[30] There was no definite cure for tuberculosis at the time, but patients could obtain some relief if they went to towns in the southwestern United States that had a high, dry outdoor climate, such as in Arizona, New Mexico, and Colorado. By using the Electropoise, people with the disease who could not afford to travel may have thought that they could receive an oxygen treatment at home without the travel or expense.

After the initial success of the Electropoise, and in an effort to better target what Sanche felt was the "right" market, he patented a new device on July 27, 1897. By 1900 the new device had become an "improved" model of Electropoise called the Oxydonor, or "giver of oxygen." The device was claimed to force oxygen into the system and

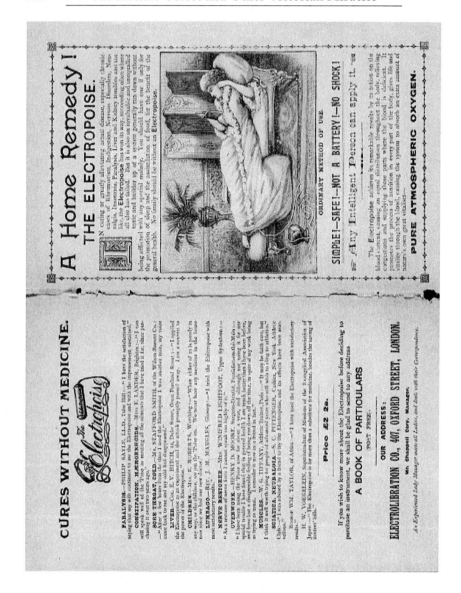

The Electropoise, later re-designed as the Oxydonor, was supposed to force healing oxygen into the system. The device was made in the shape of a sealed cylinder a little over three inches long. An attached flexible cord that came out of one end was attached to a small metal plate that was fastened to the wrist or ankle via an elastic band and buckle. When opened by scientists from the American Medical Association, the sealed metal cylinder was found to be empty (Wellcome Trust).

revitalize the blood through the pores of the skin. This improved model was a little shorter in length and, instead of being empty, contained a stick of carbon.[31] The price for the Oxydonor was now $35, instead of the original $10 for the Electropoise.

At the same time, Sanche described a mysterious "life force" called diaduction that was said to be the secret of the operation of the Oxydonor. For use, the attached metal plate was fastened to the ankle or wrist of the user, while the Oxydonor cylinder was placed in a bowl of cold water to start the generation of the diaduction force. This claimed to allow the device to force oxygen into the body. Advertising said, "It causes the whole system to be filled with oxygen from the air, eliminating disease naturally." The new device was claimed to cure all fevers, including yellow fever, within a few hours.

One particular piece of advertising for the Oxydonor contained one of the quack criteria mentioned in Chapter Two. It claimed that the device "Embodies a law of Nature unknown to medical science, but nonetheless certain in beneficial results." The name alone hinted at the might of electricity as the device was said to work through electrical power.

The user was advised to relax and lounge around reading a book during the "treatment," while the machine sent life-giving oxygen into the body. Advertising for the device depicted a typical American young woman of the Gibson Girl–type that was popular at the time, reclining on a stylish sofa and reading a novel while absorbing her oxygen.[32]

The Oxydonor had elaborate attachments known as the Animator, the Novora, the Binora, and the Vocorbis. Sanche later added the Oxydonor No. 2, with the Binora Attachment. This merely added a second ankle band and "cable" that allowed two people to receive treatment at the same time, using the same Oxydonor.

The American Medical Association was quite strong in its stance against the device, as indeed it was against other quack cures. Arthur Cramp editorialized, "that a helpless child in the throes of a fearfully dangerous—and yet, rightly treated, curable—disease, should be allowed to suffer and die because ignorant parents have been persuaded to rely on these mechanical frauds, is no less than criminal." He summed up by saying "[these devices] … are utterly worthless except as a means of enriching their exploiters."[33] Sanche resisted fraud orders from the Post Office for at least two decades.

The commercial successes of the Electropoise and the later Oxydonor were so great, and there was such a high demand for the products, that several other manufacturers quickly came out with their versions of oxygen-donor machines. Imitations were the Oxygenor, the Oxygenor King, the Duplex Oxygenator, the Oxytonor, the Oxypathor, and the Oxybon. The Oxygenor King had two cords to attach to the patient, one coming from each end of the device, one to be attached to the wrist and one to the ankle, and a control that could be moved up and down the outside of the cylinder to supposedly set the force of the device. All looked suspiciously like slight variations of Sanche's device, consisting of a metal cylinder which was empty or filled with something like sand, and with a wire that connected to a metal plate that was fastened to the ankle. Some devices had seven-inch cylinders, and some contained sulfur, charcoal, or pulverized chalk. Some had separate discs and cords for attachment to the ankle and wrist at the same time. One had interchangeable discs to treat different diseases. The cost of the various devices ranged from $25 to $35. Sanche brought legal suits against most of his competitors for patent infringement, but even the courts commented that a fraudulent device such as his should not have legal protection.

The Oxypathor, the Oxygenor, and the Oxybon all promised to improve health by increasing the body's oxygen level. The Oxypathor grandly claimed that it was a "Themo-Diamagnetic Instrument," though what that was remained unexplained. E.L. Moses of Buffalo, New York, the inventor of the Oxypathor and general manager of the company that made the device, was convicted in 1914 of using the mails for fraud. He was sentenced to eighteen months in prison for making false claims, such as the claim that the Oxypathor cured diphtheria and tuberculosis. During Moses' trial it was revealed that 5,451 Oxypathors had been sold at $35 each in three years. The manufacturing cost was estimated to be about $1.25 for each device, leaving a very large profit margin for the manufacturer.[34]

The Philadelphia Oxygenator Company made a similar device that was commonly sold from booths at local fairs. It is worth looking at a few details of their advertising because it contains several good examples of how quack companies promoted their products.

The advertising set up the problem. "For many years science has searched in vain for a perfect disease oxidizer." Then it offered the cure. "By means of the OXYGENATOR the problem is solved—great quantities of OXYGEN [capitals in the original] are induced into the human system where needed and when needed, and without cost." Even better, they took pot-shots at the competition of quack patent medicines with: "Of late years the utter fraud and worthlessness of drug medication has become more and more known, owing to the praiseworthy pioneer work done by certain magazines and other independent interests." Finally they took a negative and turned it into a positive. "All of OXYPATHY's brave fighters [i.e., their salesmen] are contending for the common good and are pledged to carry on its great work to the glorious finish. Until drug medication has been relegated to the unfortunate past, will this fight go on." This was published in the *Journal of Oxypathy*, which was conveniently published by the Oxygenator Company itself.[35] No wonder the promoters of these devices were forced out of business by the Post Office fraud division.

Similar was the Oxybon manufactured by the Oxybon Company of Chicago. Its claim was, "No Medicine! No Belt! No Battery! No Electricity!" Advertising for the Thermo-Ozone Generator, invented by S.R. Beckwith, M.D., claimed, "It is applicable to every disease, it cures most diseases in their first stage, and it cures many diseases hitherto claimed incurable."[36]

A related device was Edson's Electric Garter, which also attached to the ankle. The London Electric Fabric Company of New York advertised that its Edson Electric Garter would develop the ankle into a perfect form. This was quite exciting for males in the 1890s as women's skirts swept the ground and the ankle was one of the few parts of the female form that men occasionally glimpsed.

Radiesthesia and the Pendulum

Radiesthesia, also known as dowsing or divining, was a technique first developed in Europe in the eighteenth century for the medical diagnosis of illness. The process used a small pendulum comprised of a metal weight suspended on a chain or thread that was suspended over a patient. Without any manipulation on the part of the operator, the pendulum would, one hopes, soon begin to swing. The pattern of the swinging was supposed to indicate the patient's ailment. Supposedly the pendulum would rotate clockwise above female patients, and counter-clockwise above males, but sometimes it swung in confusing circles. The direction of rotation was not always consistent and sometimes it swung in the opposite direction, depending on the operator.[37]

In the foreword to the book *Elementary Radiesthesia and the Use of the Pendulum*, the author states, "no laboratory instrument has hitherto been devised, which has been sufficiently sensitive to record automatically the micro-waves emanating from the human cellular system." This sounds suspiciously similar to other previous forms of undetectable energy that were supposedly radiated by the human body. The author further stated that radiesthesia "is a faculty which most people possess and consists in their ability to receive rays or waves surrounding them and to pass them on, through muscular reflexes, to the instrument they are using, the pendulum."[38] The technique was supposed to be able to detect radiation emitted by a person for the diagnosis of bodily ailments; however; there was no scientific evidence that it worked. Scientific researchers claimed that in reality the movement of the pendulum was due to involuntary bodily reaction on the part of the operator.

B.J. Palmer and the Neurocalometer

Bartlett Joshua Palmer followed his father, Daniel David Palmer, into the field of chiropractic. He eventually took over his father's educational facilities and expanded them into the Palmer School of Chiropractic.

Chiropractic theory said that illness was caused by compressed nerves, which became inflamed and therefore gave off more heat than undisturbed nerves. B.J. Palmer reasoned that this heat could be measured. In 1924 he introduced the Neurocalometer, an electrical device developed by an engineer named Dossa Evins, that reportedly measured the heat released by damaged nerves and could be used to help make spinal diagnoses. The device had a probe that was moved slowly down the spine so that it could measure temperature differences radiated by the skin. The primary use for the instrument was to locate subluxations, or minor dislocations between the bones. The device was supposed to be so sensitive that it could pinpoint subluxations whether or not the patient had any symptoms.

Palmer patented the machine and made it available only to graduates of the Palmer School of Chiropractic. The device was not sold, but was leased to chiropractors for a down payment of $1,000 and monthly payments of $10 for a minimum of 10 years. The lessees' contracts with Palmer stated that they had to charge at least $10 a reading. Within a year 2,000 chiropractors had signed up. Similar competitive devices were already on the market under the names of Neurothermometer and Neuropyrometer.[39]

Another device that Palmer developed was the electroencephaloneuromentimpograph, a grand-sounding name for a complicated machine that was used before and after a spinal adjustment to show that the analysis was correct and to measure its correction. The instrument measured, evaluated, and calibrated "the quantity flow of mental impulse from brain to body, both before and after adjustment, thus proving correct place, correct time, correct manner."[40]

Radionics and the Oscilloclast

Radionics originated in California with Dr. Albert Abrams, a physician in San Francisco. Abrams received his medical degree from the University of Heidelberg in Germany in 1882, performed post-graduate studies in Europe, then returned to California to practice medicine. He became a professor of pathology at Cooper Medical College (later part of Stanford University Medical School) from 1893 to 1898. He was also the author of several reputable medical textbooks. In 1889 he was the vice-president of the California State Medical Society. By the early 1900s Abrams was a reputable expert in neurology, with a respectable background and career.

Abrams developed a method of diagnosis called spondylotherapy, his combined version of chiropractic and osteopathy, that was performed by tapping on the spine. Abrams wrote an entire book on the subject aptly titled *Spondylotherapy*, in 1910. Then he discovered that he could obtain better results if he tapped on the abdomen. He claimed that the sounds produced indicated the "vibratory rate" of a specific disease. Adams said that the "atoms of the diseased tissue produced some kind of 'radiation' that affected groups of nerve-fibers which cause muscle contractions of the abdomen wall to produce dull percussion."[41]

Over the next few years Abrams developed a system for sensing what he called the "electronic reactions" of disease and used radio waves to diagnose and cure illness. In 1916 Abrams published *New Concepts in Diagnosis and Treatment*, in which he claimed that disease was a disharmony of electronic oscillations. His theory was that all human organs, diseased or healthy, transmitted a pattern of electronic radiation or "vibrations" unique to that organ or disease, and that these frequencies could be detected and measured. He felt that healthy people radiated healthy energy, but during disease the vibrations would change to an abnormal rate and radiate frequencies that indicated illness. Every disease supposedly had a specific vibration rate that he could detect and measure with his machines. The disease could then be cured by transmitting back to the patient the same frequency as the illness, in order to neutralize the vibrations of the disease and restore equilibrium

This vibrational reading was called, somewhat grandly, after himself as E.R.A., or the "Electronic Reactions of Abrams." Abrams developed two devices. His diagnostic machine was called the Dynamizer, and the accompanying Oscilloclast cured the disease as diagnosed by the Dynamizer.

Dr. Abrams claimed that all that was needed from the patient was a drop of blood, a hair sample, or even only a handwriting sample, as these would radiate the unique "vibrational patterns" of the individual. Somewhat more suspect was that from this minute sample Abrams could also determine the subject's religion, golf handicap, gender, age, present geographical location, and foretell when the person would die. All this understandably raised controversy in the 1920s, particularly when *Scientific American* magazine of September 1924 reported that his method involved a new form of energy that could not be detected by modern instruments.[42] In hindsight this was another indicator of quack medicine.

As part of the diagnostic process using the Dynamizer, a healthy control subject had to be included in the electric circuit in order to determine the vibratory rate of the disease. The machine was connected by a wire to the forehead of the healthy individual, who stood on a grounded metal plate. A drop of blood from the ill patient was placed on a piece of white filter paper and put into the Dynamizer. The blood sample was placed in a small cup-like receptacle, or well, covered by a plate that was rubbed by the operator of the device before analysis, preferably hard enough to generate enough friction to cause a squeaking noise. Mysterious energy traveled through several complicated-looking devices, then traveled through an electrode to the healthy subject, who had to face west and be located in an area of dim light for the diagnosis to work correctly.

Abrams would then tap on (percuss) the abdomen of the healthy person. The machine picked up the vibrations and diagnosed what was wrong with the ill patient, and reported the location of the illness in the body. Rheostats (variable electrical resistors) were set to various different resistance values to tune in the vibratory disease rates. The strength of the energy was recorded in ohms. In engineering terms, the ohm is actually a measure of electrical resistance, not energy or vibration frequency. This alone would make any scientific explanation of the machine questionable.

In 1920 Abrams announced the Oscilloclast, the curing device, which was attached to patient with electrodes and transmitted vibrations for healing to neutralize disease. Oscilloclasts were leased, not sold. The lease price was $200 down and $5 a month, with lessons available at $200 for a course on how to operate it. Each machine was sealed and the lessee signed an agreement not to open it as part of their lease contract. In addition, opening it voided the warranty.

By mid–1923 more than 3,500 Abrams machines were in operation. Practitioners using his system could make between $1,000 and $2,000 a week. Seeing this, chiropractors brought out the Neurocalometer as competition.[43] In addition, Abrams developed a device called the Reflexophone, that was used for diagnosing and treating patients over the telephone.

The entire radionics scheme was another case of the fine distinction between quackery and possible misguided zeal for a new medical technique. Abrams had been a well-respected physician with an established professional reputation, therefore it was hard to disprove his

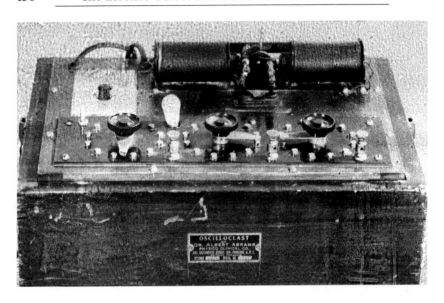

The Osciloclast was developed as one element of the diagnosis and treatments used by Dr. Albert Abrams, a physician in San Francisco, as part of his radionics system that measured vibrational readings called E.R.A., or the "Electronic Reactions of Abrams." After being attached to the patient with electrodes, this device was said to promote healing by transmitting back vibrations to neutralize the frequencies that caused illness (U.S. Food and Drug Administration: FDA 143).

claims. However, Abrams was invited by the *California State Journal of Medicine* to participate in a series of tests to determine how accurate his results were and he refused.

Being suspicious of the entire methodology, the American Medical Association and *Scientific American* magazine set up a scientific investigation of his claims. The AMA sent a specimen of blood from a healthy male guinea pig, under the name of Miss. Bell, to a practitioner in Albuquerque. The diagnosis that was returned was an infection in the left frontal sinus and a streptococcus infection of Miss. Bell's left fallopian tube. In similar fashion, a physician in Michigan sent Abrams a sample of blood from a healthy rooster, which was diagnosed as having malaria, cancer, diabetes, and two different venereal diseases.[44] A blood sample from a sheep came back with a diagnosis that said that the patient was suffering from hereditary syphilis and offered a guaranteed cure for $250. It was an intriguing mix of science, bogus theory, and questionable marketing. Some suspicious critics claimed that possibly practitioners using the devices made the patient think they had a disease and then "cured" them of something that was non-existent to begin with.[45]

After months of investigation in 1923 and 1924, *Scientific American* concluded with some understatement that the claims for the device were not substantiated and the treatments were without value.[46] As part of their investigation, scientists opened one of the sealed machines and found a disordered mix of electrical parts randomly wired together inside, but basically nothing else.[47]

The *Scientific American* investigating committee concluded that there was no such thing as "E.R.A." The *New York Times* in 1924 came out with a strongly worded editorial that Abrams was a charlatan of the first order.[48] Whatever his original motivation may have been, Dr. Abrams became very rich. When he died in 1924, he left his fortune to the Electronic Medical Foundation, which had been founded by Abrams in 1922.

Even though Abrams and his methods were discredited, his theories and similar machines did not go away. Several versions of these devices, produced by different manufacturers, were sold from the 1920s through the early 1960s. In 1940 the Art Tool and Die Co. of Detroit manufactured the Electro-Metabograph. The device was supposedly used to realign vibrations given off by diseased organs.[49] The patient was connected to the machine by two ankle electrodes which sent a series of radio signals to the patient, the specific signal depending on the illness to be cured. The FDA seized and banned the devices in 1965.

The Radioclast was manufactured by the Electronic Instrument Company of Tiffin, Ohio. Fourteen hundred of them sold for $945 each in 1942. The Homo-Vibra Ray consisted of a series of small boxes wired together, without anything inside. The Blanchard Electropathic Super Radionic Device was a similar confused mass of wiring and components. The Calbro Magnowave also supposedly tuned in on disease vibrations. The Gallert Machine was a radionics machine that sold in the 1950s for $545.

In 1954 the FDA estimated that about 5,000 related radionic devices were in use by osteopaths, chiropractors, naturopaths, and various other practitioners, and obtained an injunction against the interstate shipment of the devices.[50] In 1958, the FDA attained a permanent injunction against the interstate shipment of radionic devices. In 1961, the FDA filed criminal charges against the Electronic Medical Foundation.

We will leave the subject with this cryptic statement by the author of *Radionics*, David V. Tansley, who said in 2011, "Radionics of course is not a scientific subject in the accepted sense of the word, but this in no way invalidates its profound value to those who practice it, nor to those who receive the benefits of treatment."[51]

More Spondylotherapy

Dr. George Starr White graduated from New York Homeopathic College in 1908, and by 1915 he was a traveling salesman conducting spondylotherapy seminars for Albert Abrams. Branching out on his own, he manufactured and promoted two devices for sexual problems, the Valens Bio-Dynamic Prostatic Normalizer for treating the male prostate and rectal problems, and the Valens Bio-Dynamic Pelvic Normalizer for women. Each sold for $45. They were said to contain magnets embedded in plastic and were promoted as magnetic cures.[52]

Elements of Abrams' thinking had obviously been incorporated into White's routine as, in his diagnostic technique, the patient faced east or west while the doctor tapped/percussed the abdomen until a dull spot was found. Then the patient faced north or south and his abdomen was again percussed while he was bathed in different colored lights.

White also sold two light cures, the Rithmo-Lite Generator and the Rithmo-Chrome. The Rithmo-Lite Generator caused the light from one or more 1,500-watt lamps to fade on and off at a predetermined rate. The patient had to breathe in when the light came on and breathe out while the light went off. In other words, the light flashed on and off at the patient's rate of respiration. This was said to achieve "rhythmic harmonization of the person being treated." Respiration rate is typically sixteen to eighteen breaths per minute in adults, but this number is highly variable.

One of White's other inventions was the Filteray Pad, a patented heating pad, that was recommended for various problems, including such diverse ailments as hair loss and lumps in the breast. White encouraged using his products together, so he wanted the patient to sit on his Filteray heating pad, while being bathed with light from his Rithmo-Chrome, and breathing fumes from his Oxygen Vapor.

Drown Radiotherapy

Similar radionic therapy was championed in the 1930s by Ruth Beymer Drown of Los Angeles. She claimed that she could diagnose disease and treat it with "Drown Radio Therapy" and "Drown Radio Vision Instruments." The Drown devices and instruments were Abrams types of devices used to develop a diagnosis from a blood sample and were purported to tune in to the vibrations of the body to detect disease. Drown had another machine that supposedly broadcast healing rays to the patient by radio while they were at home. The Drown Home Radionics Device Model 98 sold for $500.

Drown published *The Theory and Technique of the Drown Radiotherapy and Radio Vision Instruments* (1939) to explain her instruments and techniques. Tests by scientists from the University of Chicago in 1947 and 1950 investigated the use of the machine, operated by Mrs. Drown herself, but failed to substantiate any of her claims.[53]

The Toftness Radiation Detector

In 1936 Irwing N. Toftness, another early follower of Dr. Abrams, began developing his own device based on Abrams' philosophy. He started with what was called the Toftness rubbing plate. It was a plate that was rubbed to produce the squeaking sound produced when practitioners rubbed the well-plate on Abrams' device.

Toftness believed that he could feel heat radiated when a subluxation or disease was present by rubbing his plate as it was held over the spine. He also thought he could feel the same heat simply by holding his hand over the patient. However, because his colleagues could not reproduce this phenomenon, he developed a device with lenses in front of the rubbing plate to supposedly amplify the heat and make it more detectable.

His first handheld device was originally called the Neurolinometer.

Over the years the design was modified and new materials were used to amplify the squeak from the rubbing plate and to give the device a more impressive look. It was marketed as the "Toftness Research Instrument" and "Toftness Radiation Detector."

Patents were issued in 1971 and 1984 for the radiation detector, which was a plastic cylinder that containing a series of plastic lenses. The device was held over a patient while the practitioner's fingers were rubbed on the top of the device in a circular manner, after the user applied baby powder to the top plastic lens. When the device was moved over a diseased part of the back, the operator's fingers would supposedly encounter increased friction and start to "stick" on the rubbing plate. The squeaks were counted. The more squeaks, the greater the nerve interference, disease, or subluxation. A lower number of squeaks indicated that the patient was beginning to improve.

Toftness opened the Toftness Postgraduate School of Chiropractic, conducted seminars on how to use the device, and leased them for use in offices. Practitioners were required to take a course for $400 and enter into a fifteen-year lease for payment of $700 for the first year and $100 for subsequent years.

Edmund S. Crelin from Yale University tested a Toftness Radiation Detector for the FDA and concluded that it was "hocus-pocus."[54] Finally, in 1982, after more than 30 years of citizens' complaints, the U.S. District Court issued an order prohibiting all use of the Toftness Radiation Detector.

In 1989, two chiropractors studied the use of a Toftness Radiation Detector to look for "upper cervical subluxations" in fifty patients. The authors concluded that the device had "fair but inadequate reliability." Not long afterward, the device was redesigned and was renamed the Sensometer.

In 1985, an article in *Today's Chiropractic* described what sounded like a similar device, the Jennetics Radiation Detector, developed by Martin Jenness.[55]

The Etheric Vibrator

Heil Eugene Crum attended the College of Drugless Physicians and emerged with several questionable degrees.[56] In 1936 he and his wife

Anna May Crum patented the Coetherator. His patent refers to the Coetherator as an "etheric vibrator" supposed to "treat human ailments by the vibration rate of ether."[57]

The device was housed in an impressive-looking wooden cabinet twenty-six inches long and eight inches or so deep and tall. The front of the cabinet contained a series of thirteen holes covered by colored discs. The main compartment inside the box contained a small light bulb that could be manually moved back and forth by a knob on the front of the box that was connected to a mechanical slider system inside. By rotating the knob, the operator moved the lamp until the desired color was illuminated. Crum claimed that he treated the patient by varying his vibration rate with the colored discs.

Part of Crum's treatment involved the patient moistening a slip of paper with saliva that was then placed into a slot in the top of the box. If saliva was not available, the practitioner could use a photograph of the patient or a specimen of his handwriting. In fact, the patient did not even have to be present, but treatments could be broadcast to them. This aspect of the "treatment" seemed to follow the Abrams method in many ways.

Crum claimed that his device could cure the usual list of ailments, such as cancer, hemorrhoids, nervous conditions, and stomach disorders. In addition, among the more unusual claims were that the patient's legs could be shortened or lengthened, dental cavities could be removed, and amputated fingers could be made to grow back into place. Among other assertions, Crum claimed that he could kill off dandelions on golf greens and fertilize fields from a distance. The courts disagreed and ruled against Crum. In 1941 the State Supreme Court of Indiana found that the device was "of no possible therapeutic value under any recognized system of treatment...."[58]

As late as the 1970s, books on the subject of radionics were still being published.[59] A book titled *Vibrations: Healing Through Color Homeopathy and Radionics* by Virginia MacIvor and Sandra LaForest was in its fifth printing in 1990. The book described in detail the use of the Pathoclast manufactured by Pathometric Laboratories of Chicago, described as being based on Abrams' earlier Oscilloclast.[60] The operator placed the patient's blood, urine, or saliva into a small test well, and then manipulated various knobs on the front panel to make a diagnosis.

Treatment was performed using the Ghadiali Spectro-Chrome color lamps, about which more will be said in Chapter Eleven.

Even in 1979 MacIvor and LaForest were still admitting that the radiation utilized by radionic instruments could not as yet be detected by using conventional scientific instruments.[61] They also admitted that controversy continued to rage over the nature of radionic energy and said, "it is indeed a field that raises new questions with every answer."[62]

One interesting point they mention is that a practitioner they discuss in detail in their book claimed that he could diagnose illness just as well with the Pathoclast instrument unplugged from the power source. Just like Abrams. The authors indicate that workers in the field "have established that the energy of the mind, rather than electronics, is the fundamental operating principle of radionics."[63]

The Harmonizer

Another curious device that used radio waves to supposedly effect a cure was the Harmonizer. The machine consisted of an AM radio, but without a loudspeaker. Instead, the audio output was connected to an electronic meter that fluctuated according to the signal when the radio was tuned to a radio station. The patient was connected to a wire that plugged into a socket that was not connected to anything inside the machine. The fluctuations of the meter while it was responding to music or speech on the radio was intended to be a visual indication to the patient that healing was taking place.[64]

NINE

Reshaping the Outside

The ideal image of the Victorian man was one with bulging muscles that were used to attract women. One of the heroes of Victorian men (and discreetly admired by the Victorian ladies) was Eugene Sandow (Friedrich Wilhelm Müeller), a German strongman and showman, sometimes nicknamed the Modern Hercules. A popular theatrical act he developed was flexing his muscles and striking dramatic poses called "muscle display performances" while wearing abbreviated clothing, in which he showed off his physique, rather than his weight-lifting ability. In an era that considered nudity to be wicked, he sometimes appeared in private sessions in only a fig-leaf, or even less, and allowed attendees to feel his well-developed, bulging muscles.[1]

The concept of being a strong muscular man was further promoted by Charles Atlas (Angelo Siciliano), a bodybuilder. His fame came from a series of cartoon-type print advertisements that started in the 1930s and continued on long after he died. These mini-dramas showed a skinny young man (usually accompanied by an attractive female companion) being threatened by a bully on the beach. The young man goes home and sends away for a free Charles Atlas training brochure. Shortly thereafter, the hero with his newly-developed muscles returns to the beach, finds the bully, gets even, and goes off with the girl. A perfect fantasy for all slightly-built young men.

One unusual way to build a better (i.e., supposedly more sexually-attractive) man was by using an odd contraption made by the Cartilage Company of Rochester, New York. Consisting primarily of a series of belts and pulleys, the machine was directed at the shorter man and was claimed to promote growth of several inches. To use the machine, one end of a rope was fastened to the head and shoulders with a series of straps. The other end of the rope was passed through a pulley fastened to a ceiling beam or other stout support. Meanwhile the feet were securely fastened to the floor by straps. Pulling on the rope to stretch the body upwards, while the feet were solidly attached to the floor, would supposedly result in a permanent height increase of several inches. Stretching exercises had to be performed twice a day for a year. At the same time this routine was claimed to broaden the shoulders and increase the chest measurements.

This dubious procedure was guaranteed to add to the height of anyone under the age of fifty by two to five inches. Interestingly most of the purchasers who gave glowing testimonials were under the age of twenty-five, at a time of life when the continued normal upward growth of childhood was to be expected.

Sold through the mail, the price of the machine was $10, though the price might be reduced to $3 as an incentive if the sales prospect did not purchase right away. The company also sold mail-order appliances to straighten bow-legs and knock-knees. A fraud order was finally issued against the company in March of 1914.[2]

Another way to build the better man was through exercise. Opportunities included calisthenics, gymnastics, boxing, fencing, wrestling, bowling, basketball, walking, golf, horseback riding, rowing, swimming, bicycling, and group games such as tennis, cricket, and baseball.

Exercising in the Bath

For those who couldn't exercise outside, other methods could be used. Early exercise machines were used for self-exercise with devices such as rowing machines and machines for lifting weights, the use of which was theorized to build muscles and release energy trapped in the body.

The Victorians loved gadgets and were very fond of bicycling as a popular way to exercise. One of the curious exercise inventions to come out of the Victorian period was the combination of a bicycle and a shower, named the velocipede-shower, invented in England and exhibited at the Paris Exhibition of 1897 as the *vélo-douche*.[3] The machine provided the means for achieving cleanliness and exercise at the same time.

The user sat on a contraption that looked like a bicycle and pedaled furiously to power a rotary pump that forced water from a tank upwards to a shower head placed above the rider. The harder the user pedaled, the more powerful the flow of water to wash him off.[4]

A earlier similar machine was Bozerian's Shower Bath from 1878, in which the pumping machinery was built into a small tub filled with water. The user stood with his feet on two small foot-rests located just above the water, and moved his weight from side-to-side on the two. One foot-rest was connected to a pump that moved the water from the tub up to a shower head positioned over the user; the other was connected to a spring that pulled the foot back down again when the weight shifted back. Thus a side-to-side rocking motion by the user kept the water continually pumping up to the shower head and then spraying down. Like the velocipede-shower, this arrangement provided exercise at the same time as a shower.

Another device that provided a workout while bathing was the "Bath Exerciser," developed by John Harvey Kellogg at the Battle Creek Sanitarium. This exercise device consisted of a metal scoop about a foot across, with handles on either side, that attached to the faucet of a bathtub by a band made of rubber tubing. The user sat in a filled tub, gripped the handles of the scoop with both hands, flexed his knees forward, and filled the scoop with water. He then straightened his legs and pulled back with a rowing motion and dumped the scoop on his chest. This action was then repeated in rapid succession for a period of five or more minutes. It was like rowing, though not moving anywhere, while using the resistance of the "oars" (the scoop) through the water to create exercise.[5]

Exercise Machines

Initially exercises were performed by the user, and included such activities as running, jumping, lifting weights, various calisthenics, and the use of Indian clubs. To provide more formal exercises, Per Henrik Ling of Sweden, an officer in the Swedish army and founder of the Royal Gymnastic Central Institute in Sweden, developed a very popular series of athletic exercises named the "Swedish Movement Cure." His system, derived from ancient Chinese exercises used for training soldiers for war, consisted of a series of gymnastic exercises that involved jumping and clapping while assuming contorted and difficult positions.

After the arrival of mechanical engines, ingenious engineers quickly adapted the use of the new steam engine and electric motor to power machines for exercising. Instead of the user exercising himself, motor-driven exercise machines at spas and sanitariums replaced active exercises with machinery that worked the muscles in various ways to perform passive exercise. The Health Lift, for example, was a weight machine that was promoted for relieving the stresses of the business life.

Ling's exercises were adapted by Gustav Zander, a Swedish physician and orthopedic specialist, for use with a series of popular machines for exercising different parts of the body. Zander's principle was to force and control the movements of the body, moving the joints to exercise each group of muscles one after the other, while measuring the amount and type of movement and the energy of every effort.

Zander used the medical gymnastics devised by Ling, but employed mechanical machines to perform the exercises. Powered by steam engines, gasoline engines, and later by electric motors, these machines forced and controlled the movement of the body to provide physical exercise. For example, his knee-flexing machine exercised the pelvis, spinal column, hips, and upper thighs. This was basically an early type of stair-stepping machine. Another example was the Zander machine used for passive conditioning of the abdomen. The machine rotated two rollers in a circle on the abdomen with a whirling, rolling, thrusting motion that was intended to strengthen the abdominal muscles.[6]

Between 1860 and 1890, Zander's exercise machinery was popular with spas, resorts, and sanitariums, all of which installed Zander machines to attract customers. Typical was the Homestead Spa in Hot Springs, Virginia, which installed thirty-six Zander machines that were used by an estimated 60,000 guests each year. Starting in 1906, free-standing Zander Institutes opened in Boston, New York, San Francisco, and Chicago.

One of Zander's more unusual exercise machines was his mechanical horse. Horseback riding and driving over rough roads had long been recommended to stimulate the abdominal muscles and overcome constipation. To mimic this motion, Zander developed a mechanical horse, called a "trotting motion" machine, to simulate riding by duplicating the movements of a moving horse. The machine, which looked somewhat like those used today by mechanical bull riders, consisted of a saddle, reins, and stirrups, and was driven by a motor connected to a drive wheel and pulley belt. The up-and-down motion of the "horse" could be adjusted to simulate various speeds and actions from a trot to a canter. The motion was designed to stimulate the digestive system during a two or three minute treatment.[7]

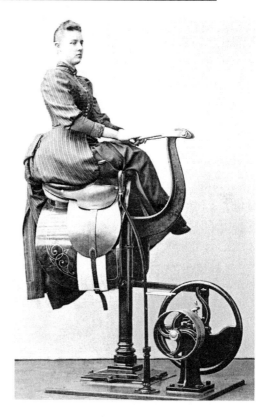

Dr. Gustav Zander of Stockholm, Sweden, designed a number of exercise machines that were powered by electric motors to exercise various muscles of the body. This motor-driven mechanical horse, called a "trotting motion" machine, duplicated the movements of a real horse to simulate the motion of riding. It was prescribed to stimulate the abdominal muscles and overcome constipation, and was also recommended as a vigorous nineteenth-century treatment for impotence in men (Library of Congress).

Vibrators for Massage

On September 4, 1821, Michael Faraday built the world's first electric motor. It was only a toy at the time and was not adapted to perform useful work for a number of years. But when it was, it opened up a host of medical applications, including the vibrator as a mechanical massage device.

Massage had long been a legitimate medical treatment for sore and aching muscles, to relax them and improve their circulation. Massage treatments varied from a mild and soothing massage with soft strokes of the fingers, to more active therapy where the body was repeatedly struck with the edge of the hand.

Effleurage consisted of mild and soothing massage with long, slow, soft strokes, with the hands, fingers, or fists. *Pétrissage* was massage with a greater degree of pressure. In *tapotement* the masseur repeatedly struck the body with the tips of the fingers or the edge of the hand. The electric vibrator was developed to provide faster and easier ways to provide mechanical massage than using these manual methods.

Electrically-powered vibrating massage machines were welcomed by the medical profession as they saved time for each treatment and removed the necessity for skilled manual labor. They performed massage treatments more rapidly and efficiently than those by hand, thus reducing the overall treatment time required and allowing more patients to be treated more effectively during a working day. Both of these, of course, equated to more money for the practitioner. The use of machine massage was a smart business decision as most massage patients neither worsened nor recovered from their condition, but required regular repeated treatments.[8] Spas and sanitariums were leading markets for early mechanized massage machines.

The use of the electrical vibrator was praised by physicians. It was considered vastly more efficient than manual massage and, by the early 1900s, mechanical massage started to replace massage performed by hand. Machine massage was more efficient than that delivered by hand and a mechanized appliance could deliver massage movements for a longer period of time than could a masseur using only the hands. A massage machine could also perform at a faster pace.

Some early massage devices were powered by a foot pedal, similar to early dental drills. One of the earliest mechanical massage devices was the "percuteur," a wind-up vibrator driven by clockwork, that was available to physicians and spas before 1870. Butler's Electro-massage Machine, sold around 1888, was a roller device that combined massage with electrotherapy.

The first electromechanical vibrator marketed to physicians was developed by British physician Joseph Mortimer Granville and manufactured by the Weiss Company. Patented in the early 1880s, the device was battery-powered and had interchangeable vibratodes, the part that applied the actual vibration through contact with the body, for application of the vibrating energy. Within fifteen years of the introduction of the first Weiss vibrator, more than a dozen manufacturers were producing both battery-powered vibrators and models that operated from line electricity.[9] Vibratodes were made of metal, wood, hard rubber, or soft rubber, and were designed in various lengths, sizes, and shapes.

Vibrating appliances for medical use were energized primarily by electric motors, but some were otherwise mechanically powered by water, compressed air, or small engines. Models of vibrating massagers varied from the Chattanooga vibrator, which was a large floor-model machine intended as a professional medical instrument that sold for about $200 in 1900, to smaller models of portable professional vibrators costing between $15 and $75, such as the Sheldon or the Wappler Electric, which were held in the hand.

Vibration could be applied to the patient in continuous or interrupted fashion, and was used either at a fixed location on the body or moved about to different locations. Vibrations were applied from slow rates of 50 to 150 strokes a minute to fast rates of several thousand per minute. The intensity of the vibrations varied anywhere from gentle stroking to deep pressure. Vibratodes were applied directly for external massage of the muscles, or to the spinal region or over the abdomen on areas over the stomach, liver, spleen, or pancreas. Vibration was claimed to be effective in either increasing or diminishing nervous sensibility, whichever was desired. Among other conditions, the Sheldon Electric Company vibrator claimed to treat asthma, dandruff, impotence, obesity, watery eyes, and wrinkles.

For general vibrotherapy to treat the entire body, the patient sat on a chair or stool, or lay on a table, that had an attached electric motor that caused the entire patient to shake. Three forms of vibration, percutient, lateral, or centrifugal motions, were used, depending on the treatment desired. The Battle Creek Vibratory Chair, for example, contained an electric motor that was attached to the seat of a chair that was mounted on coil springs. When put in motion, the chair produced violent vibrations that were supposed to improve the flow of blood and lymph to enhance cell nutrition, improve respiration, stimulate "bodily secretions," cure constipation, tone the muscles, and improve metabolism. Treatment time was usually three to five minutes. The Vibratory

Chair was manufactured by the Sanitarium and Hospital Equipment Company in Battle Creek, one of John Harvey Kellogg's many subsidiary enterprises.

The Battle Creek Sanitarium was a leading user of mechanical devices to improve health.[10] Kellogg's mechanotherapy room at the Battle Creek Sanitarium was filled with a vast collection of appliances for kneading, shaking, rubbing, and vibrating. One specialized massage treatment was called "vibration of the heart." The user stood against a round metal pad while a machine provided rhythmic punches to the chest. This treatment supposedly pushed out toxins and increased mental capacity.[11] Another specialized piece of equipment was the Bergonic Chair that a patient was strapped into and vibrated rapidly to treat cases of obesity and constipation.

Vibrators were also available for home use. White Cross Electric Vibrators were sold by direct mail order from 1902 through the 1930s, as well as through the Sears, Roebuck catalog. They provided the "Swedish Movement right in your own home." The sales emphasis was that buying your own vibrator would save money by using the device at home, instead of paying for a massage in a doctor's office. An added benefit was that this provided the privacy of self-treatment. The White Cross vibrator allegedly improved circulation and relieved ailments that had their origin in "congestion" or "poor circulation."

One of the characteristics of some quack devices to make them seem like they were doing something was to provide vibration. By jiggling the insides, vibration was one way to assure the patient that some healing treatment was being used. The Parker Vibratory Electric Bath Blanket, for example, not only warmed the body, but produced "vibratory electric effects" that promoted drugless healing, regulated the action of the heart, and equalized the circulation of the blood.

The Vibrometer and the Pulsocon

One of the more peculiar devices used for vibratory massage was the Vibrometer, invented by Dr. Garvey to apply "Dr. Garvey's System of Massage by Vibratory Motion." The device looked somewhat like a banjo, including a neck with strings on it. The device contained a motor that plucked the strings and was supposed to cure physical ailments by using the vibration rate of the musical notes.[12]

A simpler type of vibrating machine was the Pulsocon developed by Gerald Joseph Macaura, who founded a "vibrotherapy institute" in Manchester, England, in 1908, to promote the device. The machine looked like a mechanical eggbeater or an old-style manually-operated hand-drill. The user turned a crank on the side that operated gears that caused the business end of the device to pulse at up to 2,000 vibrations per minute.

The alleged benefits of using the Pulsocon were an increased circulation, loosened joints, and the elimination of chronic pain. The massager was claimed to cure pain, deafness, anemia, heart disease, cramp, polio and "women's problems."

The Pulsocon was distributed in the United States by the Cirkulon Institute of Kansas City, and sold under the Cirkulon name for $15. This was $5.50 higher than the price in England. The Pulsocon wasn't on the market for long, however, in either place. By 1912 Macaura had been charged with illegally practicing medicine in Germany and in Paris.[13]

Questionable Vibrations

Women diagnosed with hysteria were a large and lucrative market for physicians. Patients did not die and did not recover from the condition, but required regular treatments of manual stimulation to bring on the "hysterical paroxysm," the Victorian name for orgasm, to relieve their symptoms.[14] Nineteenth-century physicians found this task unpleasant and manually exhausting, and generally relegated the treatment to assistants and midwives. The Victorian male-oriented view of female sexuality was that male penetration of the female had to occur for "real" sex to take place. Because no penetration was involved in this medical treatment, physicians felt that nothing sexual was occurring when the "hysterical paroxysm" occurred.[15] Manual and mechanical stimulation for hysteria remained a part of standard medical practice until the 1920s.[16]

In 1999 a leading university press published a study by Rachel Maines titled *The Technology of Orgasm*, which offered the hypothesis that electrical vibrating massage devices were developed for genital massage of hysterical women to offer the physician a faster method of relieving their symptoms.

As might be expected, Maines' book was quickly criticized for what some critics perceived as academic shortcomings. One of the critics was Helen King, a scholar of the classics, who claimed that genital massage was not a practice of ancient medicine.[17] In addition King charged Maines with poor citation practices and the use of references that did not support her claims. Another review critical of the book was contained in a paper by Lieberman and Schatzberg, again questioning Maines' source material, though the focus of the paper was more of a critique of the peer review process in academic publication than Maines' particular subject matter.[18]

Whether or not mechanical vibrators were used for sexual purposes in the Victorian era remains a point of controversy. Possibly they were, possibly they were not, and possibly the reticence of Victorians to mention sexual activity meant that they did not mention it in specific terms. Though physician Mortimer Granville developed the first electrical vibrator, he used the device for treating neurasthenia, nerve pain, and constipation in men, and said he had never used it on hysterical women.[19]

While the details of Maine's work may be subject to critical opinion, several facts support her hypothesis (as she repeatedly states in her writing, it was a hypothesis) that vibratory devices could have been used to treat hysterical women.[20] Even if the criticisms of Maines' work have some merit, there is evidence that mechanical vibration machines could be and were used for stimulation.

Therapeutic manual manipulation had been recommended by Greek physician Galen for nuns, widows, and the chaste. In 1653, Pieter van Foreest, a prominent Dutch physician, recommended that a midwife manipulate patients to the "paroxysm" for treating womb disease. Inducement of the "spasm" thought to relieve the illness until the next session.[21]

Pelvic massage was indeed commonly recommended for patients for hysteria. Horseback riding and travel in a vibrating railway carriage were recommended as being of benefit for treating cases of hysteria. Though there were only hints on the subject, the literature on hydropathic treatments referred to the fact that pleasure could be gained in some patients by using the pelvic douche spray, which directed a high-pressure jet of water at the lower abdomen. Authors, such as leading hydropathic practitioner Mary Louise Shew, stated that this kind of hydrotherapy could produce "new and unexpected sensations."[22] Even physicians cautioned that hydrotherapy that included pulsating jets of water aimed at the abdomen should be closely supervised to prevent overindulgence.[23]

In 1869 an American physician, George Taylor, patented a steam-powered massage and vibratory apparatus that consisted of a steam-powered table with a protruding vibrating sphere that massaged the pelvic area. The device was costly, bulky, and marketed only to physicians. However, again the manufacturer warned that the treatment of female ailments should be closely supervised to prevent "overindulgence."[24]

Electrification of the home proceeded rapidly after the introduction of the electric light in 1876. The first home appliance to be electrified was the sewing machine in 1889, followed by the fan, the tea kettle, the toaster, and the vibrator in 1902. The vibrator was the fifth electrical appliance introduced into the modern home.[25]

Between about 1900 and 1920, women's magazines such as *Needlecraft, Home Needlework Journal, Modern Women, Hearst's, McClure's,* and *Woman's Home Companion* showed advertisements for home electrical appliances. Vibrators in women's magazines of the early 1900s and 1910s were marketed to women as health and relaxation aids, but advertising often contained very suggestive and ambiguous descriptions, such as the phrase "all the penetrating pleasures of youth will throb in you again."[26] In 1906 the American Vibrator Company of St. Louis, Missouri, informed women that the "American Vibrator ... can be used by yourself in the privacy of dressing room or boudoir, and furnish every woman with the essence of perpetual youth." One advertisement for the White Cross vibrator said, "All the keen relish, the pleasures of youth, will throb within you."[27] The accompanying pictures showed women applying the machines to their necks and backs, describing the feeling as "thrilling" and "invigorating." Vibrators were also marketed to men as being a nice gift for a woman, an advertising strategy that significantly was not used for toasters and tea kettles.

Advertising for vibrators disappeared from women's magazines

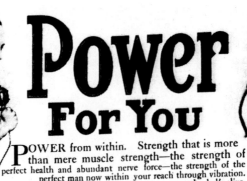

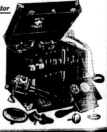

This advertisement for the White Cross Electric Vibrator explained that this was more than just a vibrator, but was a multipurpose health tool that produced galvanic and faradic electrical treatments as well as vibration. The device could even be attached to a chair to receive a "refreshing vibrating chair treatment." Similar to other vibrator advertising, this one contains the suggestive statement that "continued use over different nerve centers will bring an undeniable tingle that has not been felt in a long while" (*New York Tribune*, Jan 5, 1913).

around the end of the 1920s, about the same time that motion pictures started to show vibrators as sexual objects.[28] By the late 1920s, magazines would no longer accept advertisements for vibrators as they were concerned about violating anti-obscenity laws, and women became reluctant to purchase them because they were stigmatized as sex appliances.

Vacuum Therapy

Almost every conceivable physical measure that could be applied to the human body for a treatment has been utilized at one time or another. Acting under the assumption that constricted capillaries produced localized ailments, "the Equalizer" was an airtight device that encased various limbs (or indeed the entire body), and reduced the atmospheric pressure around the afflicted parts via a crank-driven piston. By reducing the pressure around the limb, the capillaries in the skin enlarged and delivered additional blood to the afflicted area.[29]

Blood circulation in a particular extremity could be stimulated by alternate applications of pressure and vacuum, a treatment that was recommended for many of the disturbances of the circulatory system, such as peripheral vascular disease. Typical of these devices was the Pavaex (a name derived from *passive vascular exerciser*) suction pressure boot. The limb, typically a leg, was placed inside a glass cylinder that was sealed to the upper part of the limb with a rubber cuff. Alternating vacuum and increased pressure inside the cylinder in turn attracted blood into the leg and forced it out again. Negative pressure was applied for twelve seconds, the positive pressure for three seconds.[30]

This use of vacuum technology was legitimate medical therapy. But along with the legitimate, came the questionable devices. Crosley Radio Corporation, for example, manufactured a curious baldness remedy named the Xervac starting in 1937. The concept was to use a small vacuum pump to massage the scalp by alternately using a vacuum and then slightly-increased air pressure on the head, thus allegedly stimulating hair to grow. Xervac advertising claimed, "A new scientific sensational development, XERVAC treatments will stop falling hair, will restore hair to bald heads, massages the scalp without any discomforts, no oils or tonics necessary."

The device was sold primarily to operators of barber shops and beauty parlors, and to physicians, but a smaller model was also available for home use. To apply the treatment, the user donned a metal helmet that was sealed to the head by a rubber gasket. The helmet was attached via a rubber hose to a vacuum pump that was housed in a large cabinet on the floor. The machine sold for $150, and the cost of individual treatments was $1 to $2 for a half-hour session.

Similar competitive devices were manufactured by the Modern Vacuum Pump Company of Denver and the Evans Vacuum Cap Company of St. Louis. Similar to the Xervac, both incorporated a helmet that was attached to a vacuum pump. The recommended treatment time was for fifteen minutes, twice a day.

A more complicated apparatus was the Gro-Flex. This procedure was more impressive as the user lay on a special table with their head encased in the helmet while the vacuum treatment was applied. The manufacturer claimed that "manipulating the scalp regularly will restore healthy conditions, and luxuriant hair will be the result."

Another concept

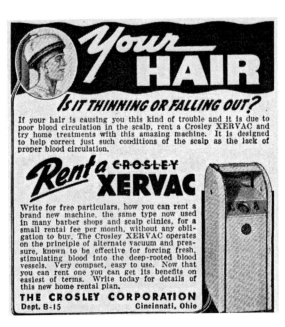

Your HAIR

IS IT THINNING OR FALLING OUT?

If your hair is causing you this kind of trouble and it is due to poor blood circulation in the scalp, rent a Crosley XERVAC and try home treatments with this amazing machine. It is designed to help correct just such conditions of the scalp as the lack of proper blood circulation.

Rent a CROSLEY XERVAC

Write for free particulars, how you can rent a brand new machine, the same type now used in many barber shops and scalp clinics, for a small rental fee per month, without any obligation to buy. The Crosley XERVAC operates on the principle of alternate vacuum and pressure, known to be effective for forcing fresh, stimulating blood into the deep-rooted blood vessels. Very compact, easy to use. Now that you can rent one you can get its benefits on easiest of terms. Write today for details of this new home rental plan.

THE CROSLEY CORPORATION
Dept. B-15   Cincinnati, Ohio

Male pattern baldness, a genetic trait passed down from an individual's parents, was a constant worry to men. One of the strange devices that promised to restore luxuriant hair was the Xervac. The concept was to use a small pump to massage the scalp by alternately using a vacuum and then a slightly-increased air pressure on the head, thus allegedly making hair grow. As shown in this 1940 advertisement from the manufacturer, the user donned a metal helmet that was sealed to the head by a rubber gasket and attached via a rubber hose to a vacuum pump that was housed in a large cabinet on the floor (author's collection).

for growing hair was the Thermocap, made by Allied Merke Institutes of New York City. To quote the manufacturer: "The Thermocap Treatment is entirely different from anything known or used in this country before." The treatment ("...as soothing and restful as an afternoon nap") consisted of placing the Thermocap (which looked somewhat like a fez) on top of the head, attaching it to a source of power and heating up the scalp for ten minutes every day. The heat source was a light bulb, but it was supposed to irradiate the top of the head with "blue light from a special actinic quartz ray bulb."[31] The user was instructed to place the cap on his head for a few minutes whenever he had time, plug the power cord into a wall socket, and the Thermocap would send just the correct amount of heat into the scalp to stimulate hair growth.[32]

The manufacturer of the Thermocap claimed that for men and women with falling hair it would not only produce "...beautifully thick, luxuriant hair that is the admiration of all their friends," but "... in the great majority of cases, would actually grow hair on heads *that were even completely bald*" [italics in the original]. One satisfied user claimed, "My hair is growing so fast that each hair seems to be running a race with its brothers and sisters, to see who will get there first."[33]

Reshape Your Nose at Home

Devices for re-forming the nose became popular in the 1930s for those who were dissatisfied with their outward appearance. Basically these devices were all the same. They consisted of a metal housing that fitted over the nose, then utilized several adjustment screws to force the nose into the desired shape.

One of these devices was the Trados Model 25 New Nose Shaper. Made from brass, the device fitted over the nose and contained five metal plates that were adjusted via equalizing screws. The idea was that pushing hard enough on the nose over a long time with the plates would eventually realign the entire structure. However, users were cautioned to only adjust the device very slightly during treatment to avoid damage to their noses.

A similar device called the Sculptron was a metal cover intended to straighten the nose. Originally selling for $6, the price eventually declined to $2 to match the hard economic times of the Great Depression. Nevertheless, the company sold 800,000 of their nose reshaping devices before being shut down by the Post Office.

Another nose shaper was the Model 25 Trilety Nose Straightener. The Trilety promised "to improve the shape of your nose by remolding the cartilage and fleshy parts, quickly, safely, and painlessly, or refund your money." The Anita Nose Adjuster was advertised to adjust your nose while you slept.

Medical Implications of Women's Corsets

A popular fashion trend in the Victorian era was the re-shaping of women's bodies through the use of corsets. The second half of the nineteenth century saw a rise in the use of tightly-laced corsets for women, and the manufacture of corsets became a thriving industry. Though corsets are not generally considered to be a medical device in themselves, the wearing of corsets by Victorian women to reshape their figures caused various medical problems.

Corsets were used by the ancient Greeks and Romans, but they disappeared during the Dark Ages, and did not re-appear until the late Middle Ages. In the sixteenth century, Queen Elizabeth I of England liked to show off her very fashionable corseted figure.[34]

The stiffening material of a corset, the straight vertical strips that gave a corset its power and shape, were called busks or stays. In the seventeenth and eighteenth centuries, bone, stiffened leather, and wooden stays were gradually replaced by ones made of iron and steel, and what was called whalebone, thought the whalebone in corsets was actually baleen, a stiff flexible substance that grows from the upper jaw of certain whales. The corset itself eventually became laced up the back, requiring assistance with tightening the laces, and had strong hooks down the front. Nineteenth-century Victorian corset technology involved lacing that was designed with the latest mechanical engineering principles for additional tightening power, with strong metal catches for the fasteners.

The Victorian era was the age when the perfect example of femininity was a well-shaped figure with a tiny waist, a large bosom, and hefty hips. A well-developed chest was considered to be an indication of a naturally vigorous constitution and the ideal for the proper breeding of families. Below the waist, wide hips and thick, sturdy legs were considered to be the perfect shape for good child-bearing.[35] The ideal figure was an hourglass shape with a wasp-waist created by tightly-laced whalebone corsets. This hourglass shape was called the "French" shape. A corset forced a woman to have a tantalizingly small waist, while being pleasingly plump above and below.

Husbands were supposed to be able to span their wife's waist with their two hands. Therefore a twenty or twenty-one inch waist was considered to be perfect. One measure was that an appropriate waist size for a woman should be the same as her age when she married, and most women intended to be married before age twenty-one.[36] With continued pressure produced by a tightly-laced corset, some women forced their figures to have what they considered to be an ideal nineteen-inch waist circumference.

Doctors, however, warned that the practice of tight-lacing of corsets could lead to problems with the lungs, stomach, and reproductive organs.[37] Even in the seventeenth and eighteenth centuries, physicians were warning against the practice of tight corseting. One of the earliest known medical warnings about corsets appeared in 1602 from physician Felix Plater.[38] Medical opinion, however, was contradictory. Not all physicians were against corseting, and some continued to promote their use, in spite of the known dangers.[39]

The most common complaint of physicians dealing with corseted women was an injury that was referred to as "chicken breast," a condition where the extreme pressure of some tightly-laced corsets turned the lower ribs inward so far that it caused them to overlap due to the continual pressure. Ribs could also ride up over the sternum (breastbone) and fracture. The lower (or vertebral) ribs, the so-called "floating ribs," which are not attached to the breastbone, were most at risk for this injury. There were anecdotal stories that to prevent this and enhance their tiny waists, some women actually had the lowest ribs on each side surgically removed in their quest for what they perceived to be "the perfect figure." This, however, is difficult to document and seems unlikely in light of the dangers of surgery that were prevalent at the time.

In any case, the pressure on the ribs caused an inability to breathe properly, which in turn caused insufficient respiration, fractured ribs,

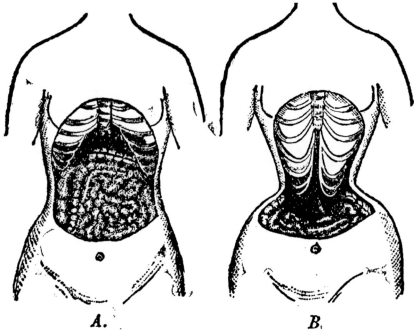

A.   *B.*

lbs of large curve; the lungs large   The ribs bent almost to angles
my; the liver, stomach and bow-   lungs contracted; the liver, stomac
their normal position; all with   intestines forced down into the p
nt room.   crowding the womb seriously.

Nature versus Corsets, Illustrated.

The dangers of corseting are shown by comparing these two illustrations. The drawing on the left shows a woman's outline before the use of a corset. The ribs and lungs, along with the viscera, including liver and intestines, are in their natural positions. In the drawing on the right, after corseting, the ribs have been compressed to the point of overlap, limiting the expansion of the lungs. The stomach, liver, and intestines have been forced down into the pelvis, and are pressing hard on the other internal organs, including the uterus (Library of Congress).

and injuries to the sternum and clavicle. The loss of breathing capacity was actually measured by one scientist, and the average reduction was about 20 percent.[40] The lungs in the areas of compression sometimes atrophied and collapsed. One eminent physician even suggested that use of the corset might lead to a high incidence of tuberculosis and other diseases of the chest among women, due to an inadequate ability to breathe properly.[41]

Even though some of these problems were known, upper and

middle-class women still continued the practice of tight-lacing, as fashion dictated that they have an hourglass figure that was supposed to be attractive to men. Though wearing corsets has been attributed mostly to upper-class Victorian women, fashion historians have shown that working-class women also considered corsets to be an essential part of their daily dress, if for no other reason than they wanted to emulate their employers and social betters.

Ironically, though, what was supposed to be creating a sexually attractive figure was causing damage in the name of fashion. Pressure was exerted upwards on the lungs, stomach, and heart. The constant pressure from the corset caused some of these internal organs to be forced up into the chest and throat, and others downwards into the pelvic area, resulting in chronic suffering from weak backs and disturbances of the internal organs. One of the injuries reported was "tight-lace liver," which was compression of the waist to the point where the liver became damaged.[42]

Even though women complained about the brutality of tightly-laced corsets, they continued to use them, many of them to please their husbands.[43] Another of the appeals was that a corset gave the appearance of fashionable aristocratic leisure. A woman could not conveniently stoop, bend over, pick up things from the floor, or exercise, inferring that she had no need to perform these tasks. She could stand or sit, but most women with tight corsets frequently had difficulty breathing while doing so. Not surprisingly, women who wore tight corsets commented on a choking sensation and inability to breathe properly, hence the popular Victorian piece of furniture, the fainting couch, for sudden unexpected collapses.

A particularly undesirable by-product of tightly-laced corsets used to achieve an hour-glass shaped figure was that the garment placed tremendous downward pressure on the abdomen and pelvic organs. By the 1860s, many physicians were warning that corsets compressed the reproductive organs and weakened a woman's ability to bear healthy children. Some physicians felt that physical characteristics could be inherited and feared that a deformed waist from corseting could be inherited and the trait transmitted to their future offspring.[44]

Contemporary medical writings showed that there was a definite relationship between constricting corsets and "female complaints." A few enlightened physicians confirmed that pressure on the abdomen from wearing tight corsets resulted in a variety of physical illnesses, ranging from nausea, a lack of appetite, headaches, constipation, disrupted menstrual cycles, fainting due to difficulty in breathing, and the most serious, uterine displacement.

Miscarriages were sometimes deliberately induced by wearing tightly-laced corsets. This use of tight corsets allowed women to convince themselves that they had never really been pregnant in the first place and that the "obstruction" had finally cleared itself. Wearing tight corsets by pregnant women resulted in miscarriages, stillborn babies, malformed infants, and a high rate of mortality among fetuses that successfully survived to birth. Physician Alice Stockham wrote in 1883 that the direct cause of these problems was a lack of oxygen delivered to the fetus because constricting corsets inhibited the mother's breathing. Stockham stated quite bluntly, "tight lacing [was] the chief cause of infant mortality."[45]

Pressure on the liver, stomach, small intestines, and large intestine created a sense of uneasiness, a sense of pelvic weight, back pain, and aching of the inner thighs. Other symptoms included a pale complexion, palpitations, loss of breath upon exertion, swollen legs at the end of the day, and "bilious attacks." These problems did not appear in men or thin women, and were relieved (not surprisingly) by bed rest or at night, when the corset was not worn, though many physicians did not make the connection.[46] The use of the corset was blamed for every ailment from hepatitis, liver problems, and cancer, to red noses, wrinkles, clumsiness, and apathy.[47] Phrenologist Orson Fowler, author of a pamphlet-sized booklet with the long-winded title, *Tight-Lacing, Founded on Physiology and Phrenology; or, the Evils Inflicted on Mind and Body by Compressing the Organs of Animal Life, and Thereby Retarding and Enfeebling the Vital Functions*, claimed that the use of corsets would force a woman's blood into the abdomen and thus inflame "amative desires."[48]

The corset was correctly blamed for uterine congestion, due to the tight binding. One of the serious problems was the tendency to induce a sagging or prolapsed uterus, or falling of the womb. The uterus collapsed and was forced out of place, and slid down into the vagina due to the pressure. The condition was made worse by advancing age and the birth of numerous children. Treatment included support for the womb with wood, ivory, bone, rubber, ceramic, metal, or glass pessaries, mechanical devices that were inserted into the vagina to hold the uterus in place after it became displaced. These uterine supports were worn internally and held in place in the vagina by a waistband. Between 1850 and 1885 at least twenty-six different designs of pessaries were patented.[49]

Other remedies included sponges for support and the application of faradic current from a medical battery to strengthen the muscles. Doctors seeking a female clientele often advertised that they supplied a wide range of "supporting devices." However, use of these devices could lead to further "female problems" due to infection or damage to internal organs. Promoting what would appear to be contradictory goals, several proprietary designs of corset were available with a built-in pessary, so that the corset was tightly-laced and pushed the uterus downwards, while the pessary attempted to push it back up again.

Tightly-laced corsets started to go out of fashion in the early 1900s. Corsets became even lighter and looser and their use diminished drastically by the early 1910s as unrestricted fashions became an expression of the new woman's freedoms. Bloomers, corsets, and thick black stockings were replaced by loose silk clothing. By the 1920s the new fashion trend was a boyish flapper look for women that did not emphasize the waistline or chest. Ironically a contributing factor to the end to the corset era came with the beginning of World War I in 1914, when the steel that was used for stays was diverted instead to build battleships.[50] Women reportedly also donated the metal strips from their corsets. Anecdotal estimates are that enough was donated to build two battleships.[51]

Bust Developers

Women's shapes have always been subject to alteration, depending on the dictates of fashion at any particular time. In the late Victorian Age the ideal shape for a woman was a big bust and large hips. This showed that the successful husband, who was typically on the plump side also, could afford to support a wife in style with plenty of food. By the flapper era in the 1920s and the boyish look, a flat chest was considered to be fashionable and desirable, and women wore under-garments that flattened the chest. Interestingly, the two eras with such extremes in male tastes followed each other very closely in time.

Bust size has always been a subject of considerable interest to American men. However, there is no known exercise program, diet, herbal medicine, ointment, or machine that is known to be able to increase bust size, though it has been a desired goal for some for a long time. Methods tried included massage, creams, electricity, vacuum appliances, and the use of drugs. The only reliable method to increase flat chests was to use a padded corset insert, which was common in the late 1800s and has lasted until today. The basic design was a shaped piece of material with pockets into which pads of various sizes could be placed.

However, hope always springs eternal and a variety of quack treatments were sold to hopeful young women. One method that has been consistently used to try to increase bust size is some form of vacuum device to promote the health and shape of what the sales staff felt were idea breasts. Typically a soft rubber cup was placed over each breast, and the air exhausted with a vacuum pump. The concept was loosely associated with the practice of cupping to draw blood to the skin. The assumption was that it was beneficial to draw blood from the internal organs to the surface of the skin in order to cause better blood flow in the chest.

One such device was the Allure Bust Developer. It was housed in an appealing pink metal case that contained a pump to produce a vacuum. Two soft cups, attached to flexible tubing that was connected to the vacuum pump, were placed over the breasts and the vacuum initiated to supposedly enlarge them. The FDA ordered the machines destroyed in late 1950s.

Similar breast enlarger vacuum pumps used foot and hand power to create the vacuum. The earlier Abunda Beauty bust developer ($29.95) in the late 1950s was water powered and attached to a faucet with running water to create the vacuum. The FDA seized the devices in 1960 after their investigation showed that the Abunda Beauty did not meet any of its promises. The Lady Bountiful enlarger from Hollywood also used water power to create a vacuum. Such devices continued to appear into the 1970s.

Electric Body Toning

Electronic muscle stimulators (EMS) supposedly "exercised" muscles by jolting them with enough electricity to cause involuntary muscle contractions. Electronic muscle stimulators promised to do all the exercising necessary to remain healthy. Similar to the electrical treatments of 1900, these devices applied electrical currents to the muscles, causing them to contract, and thus supposedly exercising them. They were promoted for body toning, weight loss, wrinkle removal, cellulite removal, and bust development.

One such device was the Relaxacizor. The user placed contact pads at various locations on the body where he (or more typically she) wanted to remove fat. The device sent a low-level electrical current into the skin that was supposed to contract muscles, making them firmer and the user slimmer.[52] Supposedly an hour with the Relaxacizor spent reading a book, smoking, or dozing, was the equivalent of a five-mile walk or a round of golf. Over 400,000 Relaxacizors were sold between 1949 and 1970 before a federal judge ruled that the device was capable of aggravating many medical problems, causing others, and even causing possible heart failure.[53]

The Roll-a-Ray was a massager manufactured by O.A. Sutton Company around 1940 that provided infrared heating during a massage. According to their advertising, the combination of the rubber rollers and the infrared radiation was intended to "melt away" excess flab.

One of the more recent devices was the Nemectron apparatus for bio-electric treatments, which was also claimed to be effective in increasing or reducing bust size. Among its proclaimed benefits was effectiveness in regenerating the tissues, rejuvenating the nerves, overcoming the ravages of age, restoring the elasticity of the skin, and removing wrinkles and double chins, thus producing a younger-looking appearance in users by toning the body. Voltage was applied to the body part via four applicator pads. In 1959 the FDA decided that labeling for the device contained false and misleading representations of the effectiveness of the various benefits the device was supposed to offer.[54]

In 1996, the FDA determined that the Executive Briefcase from Executive Fitness Products could also cause irregularities in heart rhythm, and ordered the machines destroyed.

TEN

Treating the Insides

Before the late nineteenth century, one of the few ways to treat the abdomen and the insides of the human body without performing risky surgery was to pound, knead, bathe, and massage the contents from the outside. The reason for this was that until the appropriate sterile techniques for surgery had been developed, the inside of the body was generally inaccessible to physicians. The risk of drastic abdominal surgery was far too great for any less than life-saving treatments. Before the use of anesthesia was safe and effective, both doctor and patient viewed abdominal surgery as a last resort. It was typical for both to wait until an illness had developed to a very serious point before the patient would agree to be cut open. Very little could be done with the gallbladder, kidneys, liver, or similar internal components, though the urinary bladder could be accessed via the urethra. The other way was to treat the internal system was through natural body openings, either through the mouth at the top end of the gastrointestinal tract or via the anus at the bottom end.

At the same time, Americans, along with the British and other Europeans, had long been obsessed with their bowels.[1] Two relatively minor chronic gastrointestinal ailments that were the objects of many treatments in Victorian society were dyspepsia (indigestion) on the upper end of the digestive tract and costiveness (constipation) on the lower. Both were often the result of poor diet, the excessive use of alcohol, and reckless overeating, all of which were common practices at the time. Both ailments were common, though not fatal, diseases and as such were often ideal targets for the types of treatments offered by both quacks and established medicine. For example, the popularity of Victorian spas and spa treatments, which included drinking dreadful-tasting mineral spring water, was part of a more general concern of ridding the body of disease by easing dyspepsia and constipation.

Dyspepsia, or indigestion as it is now better known, was an important and much-discussed topic in America in the early 1830s. Dyspepsia was not a disease in itself, but was a symptom of other internal disorders. Typical symptoms were stomach pain, nausea, heartburn, acid reflux, painful belching, and flatulence.

The two primary causes of dyspepsia for Americans in the eighteenth century and early nineteenth century were poor eating habits and the excessive use of alcohol. Over-eating, and the resulting excess weight gain, led to widespread stomach troubles that plagued nineteenth-century Americans to the point where the 1800s were known as the era of "The Great American Stomach Ache."[2]

Constipation has always been an indelicate subject. Discussion or jokes about it are considered childish or distasteful, though it is prominent in the medical literature and in popular culture.[3] Medical anxiety about the perceived dreadful consequences of constipation increased through the late 1800s and early 1900s. As late as 1932, the stated opinion of physician William Kerr Russell was, "There is no doubt at all that constipation is a most potent cause of a great deal of human suffering; it probably is indirectly responsible for more misery than many of the so-called killing diseases."[4] Another sinister-minded American health writer even stated darkly that constipation could result in pressure on the nerves, resulting in mental dysfunction, which might lead the sufferer to commit arson, robbery, murder, or other crimes. Other writers agreed with him.[5]

Health reformers, entrepreneurs, and quacks put forward an astonishing variety of preventives and remedies for this ancient dreaded affliction. Victorian spas and sanitariums around the turn of the twentieth century treated a variety of medical ailments, but particularly dyspepsia, constipation, and neurasthenia. As John Harvey Kellogg, superintendent of the world-renowned Battle Creek Sanitarium put it, "Most of the patrons of the institution are persons who are suffering from chronic disease, especially gastric and nervous disorders."[6] Under his supervision, the sanitarium attracted wealthy and middle-class residents who had convinced themselves that dyspepsia and constipation put a damper on their ability to advance socially, professionally, and economically. The dread among the public peaked in the 1910s and 1920s with the fears of autointoxication described later in this chapter. After valiant efforts by physicians to treat the bowels with all manner of electrical and mechanical means, their enthusiasm shifted in focus in the early 1900s with the development and widespread use of new laxative drugs and better theories about disease.

As a better understanding of the causes of disease was gained, new methods of medical treatment started to develop, along with the growth of physician specialization and the complex instrumentation and technology that make up modern medicine. Even through these changes occurred, an obsessive focus on the bowels remained. Physical culture expert Bernarr McFadden believed in extreme physical exercise to prevent constipation. One of his preventive recommendations was to slap the abdominal muscles for five to ten minutes to stimulate and strengthen them. Another, more curious, method he recommended was to swallow three to six teaspoons of sand every day.[7] One simple method recommended for massage of the colon was to lie down and place a small cannonball, weighing about twenty to twenty-five pounds, on the abdomen, and then roll it around over the pathway of the colon underneath.[8]

The concept of massage to prevent constipation led to the use of various mechanical devices to knead, vibrate, and pound the abdominal muscles. One English physician believed in various types of massage and percussion applied to the lower spine, buttocks, and abdomen to stimulate the defecation reflex. Another treatment used a special vibrating chair that shook the patient rapidly up and down. Yet another used a table on which the patient lay face down twice a day, while six mechanical arms on the surface of the table moved back and forth in succession to produce a rotary kneading motion around and around the abdomen in circular treatment for fifteen to twenty minutes.[9] One particular model of Zander exercise machine had two rollers that rotated in a circle around the abdomen with a whirling, rolling, thrusting motion that was intended to strengthen the abdominal muscles.[10]

A similar, but manually-operated, abdominal massage machine was the Kolon-Motor, a device that attached to the wall and had a rounded projection that pulsed the abdomen when the user turned crank handles mounted on the sides of the device. This abdominal massage was supposed to stimulate the bowel as a cure for constipation and autointoxication. The device could also be used on the lower back to stimulate the nerves. Abdominal massage given by these machines was supposed to make users feel like they were undergoing a scientific form of massage treatment, rather than that obtained via the usual manual methods.

Another peculiar technique employed by legitimate physicians to relieve constipation was the insertion of a small rubber balloon into the rectum. When it was in place, it was inflated with air or water and left in place as long as required.[11] A similar device was also used to perform a type of internal intestinal massage. After the balloon was inserted, it was alternately slowly inflated and then deflated four to six times a minute, for five to ten minutes, to produce a massaging effect from the inside.[12]

Though these methods were used by well-meaning physicians, some seem downright bizarre. For example, the use of Klemm's Muscle Beater, which consisted of a series of steel springs attached to a handle that was used to beat and batter the abdomen to stimulate the internal muscles. A similar device for the same purpose was constructed with rubber balls on the end of flexible rods that were joined at the other end to form a handle. The massage hammer, used in the same way, had a head made of soft rubber attached to a handle just like a domestic hammer for driving nails. The focus of all these devices was to stimulate the abdominal muscles into intestinal activity through brute force.

Catering to the obsessive desire of some physicians to do anything they could to empty the bowels, some models of vibrator, such as the Physician's Vibragenitant, manufactured by Gorman, had a special soft, flexible, rubber vibratode that was inserted five to six inches into the rectum and then vibrated for three to five minutes to try to stimulate the bowels into action. For stubborn cases, the physician might use a fifteen-inch flexible rubber vibratode. One variation was to use a two-foot-long soft rubber tube that was inserted into the rectum to inject a quart or more of warm water into the lower bowel while simultaneously vibrating the tube to provide stimulation of the intestines.[13]

Similar treatments were recommended for men for enlarged prostates and prostatitis. For women, vibratodes were inserted into the vagina to perform vibratory treatments of rectoceles, cystoceles, relaxed walls, and vaginismus.[14]

Shocking Treatments

Much of the focus of electrical treatments was on administering to the bowels, and rectal electrodes were supplied as standard accessories for medical batteries and electrical generators. Electrotherapists were all in favor of this. In 1909 gastroenterologist Samuel Gant said, "...at the present writing electrotherapeutists in general concede that nearly all forms of electricity are a valuable aid in overcoming sluggishness of the bowel." He added, "Another advantage of electricity is that it frequently appeals to the patient, makes him feel that something definite is being done, and enables the attendant to manage him while the other necessary steps to effect a cure are being carried out."[15] This would appear to be a definite endorsement of the placebo effect.

Electricity was used to stimulate the bowel in several ways. One was with the placement of one of the electrodes on the abdomen and the other on the lower back and then applying galvanic (continuous) stimulation between the two. With the electric current flowing, the electrode at the front was moved around the external abdomen over the area of the colon to induce contractions of the abdominal muscles. For an extra jolt, both galvanic and faradic current might be used at the same time. If this procedure failed, one of the electrodes was inserted into the rectum and electric current applied in a treatment called "faradization of the rectum."[16]

The most powerful electrical treatment of the bowels was the application of electric current combined with an enema, in a procedure sometimes called "electro-enteroclysis" or an "electric enema." The practitioner inserted a rubber tube or a special flexible irrigating electrode into the patient's rectum and injected a quart or so of saline solution. Thus the fluid-filled lower bowel in essence became one of the electrodes, in order to carry current throughout the entire lower colon. The other electrode, in the form of a flat plate, was placed on the back next to the spine or on the belly button, or moved over the external surface of the lower abdomen while electric current was passed between the two. The treatment typically lasted from ten to twenty minutes, daily at first, then reduced to every two or three days.[17] With what would seem like understatement, one practitioner commented, "The patient should not experience more than a distinct, slightly painful prickling sensation."[18]

Autointoxication

The idea of ridding the body of toxic substances was certainly not a new one. Mankind has had a morbid obsession with the products of elimination of the human body since before recorded history. In the fourth century BC, Greek physician Herodotus, who traveled extensively in ancient Egypt, noted that the Egyptians fasted and used purgatives, clysters, and emetics for three consecutive days of each month in the belief that illness had its roots in the food they consumed.[19]

Greek physicians observed that sickness was often accompanied by vomiting, profuse sweating, and violent bowel actions, and reasoned that this was the way the body was trying to purge itself of the illness. Further reasoning assumed that if these bodily actions could be induced during an illness, then the illness could be cured. Therefore, much of pre–nineteenth-century medicine was devoted to producing these actions. Seventeenth-century physicians were so obsessed with emptying the bowels that the era has sometimes been nicknamed the "age of clysters." The medical obsession for treating the bowels rose to a frenzy during the late 1800s with a new theory called autointoxication.

The basic scientific work that explained how germs caused disease was performed by French chemist Louis Pasteur and German physician Robert Koch in the 1860s and 1870s. Over the next twenty years, the causes of most infectious diseases were discovered and by 1895, in an excess of zeal, germs were being blamed for everything. After the germ theory was accepted, the Egyptian concept of retained residues of food as the cause of illness received new scrutiny and led to a widespread belief in the theory of autointoxication. This was the name used to describe self-poisoning from retained bacteria within the body, or self-poisoning arising from the intestinal tract.

Constipation now received a new lease in life under the general heading of "autointoxication," which was considered to be a serious and scientific diagnosis because it incorporated the new germ theory. Early impetus for what eventually became a new obsession with the bowels came from the work of Charles Bouchard, an eminent medical authority and professor of pathology in Paris, who was the first to coin the term "autointoxication" and was considered to be the primary authority on the subject in the 1880s.[20] The theory was that when waste material collected in the bowel, various toxic chemicals were absorbed into the body through the lining of the colon. Bouchard and other physicians noted that the retention of "poisonous products" (i.e., constipation) was often accompanied by vague symptoms, such as headache, indigestion, insomnia, nervousness, poor appetite, impotence, and physical and mental lethargy.

Radical as it was, this theory was widely accepted by the medical profession and, by 1890, autointoxication had become an important element of American health ideas. Intuitively it had made sense, and it appeared now to be proven by the new science of bacteriology.[21]

Physicians noted that constipation was a frequent complaint of patients who appeared to have no definite organic cause of illness. Previously these patients had often been vaguely diagnosed as suffering from neurasthenia. Physicians noted that many of the "manifestations of chronic intestinal autointoxication" sounded like the equally vague symptoms of neurasthenia, seemingly confirming the link between the two. Given the new thinking on autointoxication, it seemed simple and logical, then, to now diagnose neurasthenic patients as suffering from autointoxication.[22] Autointoxication became the new catch-all diagnosis for functional disorders of indeterminate origin.

The theory of autointoxication was further popularized by Nobel Prize winner Élie Metchnikoff, a respected and reputable scientist, and former deputy director of the Pasteur Institute in Paris. In later life Metchnikoff became concerned with his own mortality and shifted his focus of study to that area. Even though no scientist had proven that the products of the human intestine were able to cause any harm, Metchnikoff claimed, "Not only is there auto-intoxication from the microbial poisons absorbed in cases of constipation, but microbes themselves may pass through the walls of the intestines and enter the blood."[23]

Support for the autointoxication theory also came from eminent British physician William Arbuthnot Lane, a surgeon and member of the Royal College of Surgeons. Lane came to believe that the colon developed unnatural kinks that contributed to intestinal slowdown (stasis) and constipation, and he developed a surgical method for removing them.[24] He even said that autointoxication "is the cause of all the chronic diseases of civilization, I have no doubt."[25] Lane identified what he thought was a particularly problematic section of the bowel that became known as "Lane's Kink." Lane specialized in surgically removing this kink to "correct the often fatal consequences of autointoxication."[26]

Lane also felt that tight lacing of corsets contributed to this kinking (and hence constipation), because corsets pushed the viscera down into the pelvis. Indeed, tight lacing had been given as a cause of constipation in the late 1800s and one enthusiastic critic even suggested that it was the cause of the death of "thousands."[27]

Noted authority Samuel Gant said, "Furthermore, the colon seems to be the place for the absorption of toxic substances developing in the course of abnormal decomposition of proteins. ... This so-called auto-intoxication is becoming more and more generally recognized as a cause of certain obscure diseases."[28]

Specialist Alcinous Jamison put it even more strongly: "We are a nation of constipated people, so constipated indeed that we have developed dyspepsia and neurasthenia. As I have already stated, the chief ill of 'civilized' people is proctitis [chronic inflammation of the rectum and anus]; the chief symptom of proctitis is constipation; the chief symptom of constipation is dyspepsia; and the chief symptom of dyspepsia is neurasthenia, and so on and on—all of them the outcome of imperfect elimination of morbid matter from the intestinal canal."[29] William Kerr Russell stated, "It is, however, obvious that chronic stagnation of the bowels must lead to a chronic poisoning of the whole system."[30]

As a result, "autointoxication" became the new prestige diagnosis. As advances in science and medicine discovered more about the inner workings of the body and digestion, some of the autointoxication theory was found to possibly have a vague basis in practice, thus seeming to confirm the diagnosis and therefore increase its popularity. Indeed, the decomposition of residual protein in the diet by bacteria in the intestines resulted in chemical compounds that were present in human feces which smelled unpleasant or were toxic. Physicians looked on this as confirmation of their suspicions that the human bowel contents were deadly and that the body could poison itself by absorbing products of putrefaction from the colon.[31] The idea seemed to be confirmed by the fact that excrement was dangerous, as deadly diseases such as cholera and typhoid were spread by food and water contaminated by improper disposal of sewage.

Thus, from approximately 1900 to 1940 the threat of autointoxication from retained body waste motivated the public to partake in a remarkable assortment of anti-constipation measures.

The Professional Irrigators

The autointoxication concept became so popular that many physicians re-designed their offices to treat the many patients who were now being diagnosed with the problem. Many of the usual methods were employed, starting with vibration treatments. Samuel Gant said, "In intestinal auto-intoxication the condition of the patient can be rapidly improved through direct vibratory stimulation applied to the lymphatic glands, skin, kidneys, liver, spleen, and intestine."[32]

Gant also recommended that the attending physician should have a conveniently located hydrotherapy establishment and irrigating room with toilet facilities, as well as vibrators and a complete outfit to effectively apply water to the skin, hollow viscera, stomach, colon, and rectum. Kellogg's response to autointoxication at the Battle Creek Sanitarium was to make extensive therapeutic use of enemas and to heavily promote colonic hydrotherapy in the United States. He recommended intestinal lavage for almost all his patients.[33]

One of the popular treatments at nearly all spas and sanitariums in the United States, Europe, and the rest of the world in the late 1800s and early 1900s was internal bathing to combat neurasthenia and autointoxication. Spa physicians continued the tradition of Heroic Medicine of purging, but instead of using toxic drugs such as calomel, they accomplished the same objective with enemas and other mechanical forms of internal irrigation, which came to be thought of as the most direct and natural method of keeping the bowels pure and the body healthy.

Colonic irrigation, or the repeated washing out of the large intestine by the introduction of a long rubber tube and flushing with water, started at spas and sanitariums at the end of the nineteenth century, particularly in Germany and the United States. Physicians at the Victorian spas of the late 1800s in Germany, Austria, France, and Switzerland expanded on these earlier ideas and took them to even higher levels with a new series of treatments, vigorously washing out the insides of dyspeptic, neurasthenic, and overweight patients in the name of better health. By the late 1800s, spas and sanitariums centered much of their treatment around lavage of the colon, and almost all spas had colonic hydrotherapy departments to perform irrigation using their own local mineral waters.

To remove the unpleasant connotations that many people associated with the word "enema," the procedure was typically referred to by the politer and more neutral name of Plombières Douche. Other common names were internal bathing, or intestinal lavage. The Plombières Douche became popular because of Arbuthnot Lane and autointoxication theories. It was heavily promoted by spa physicians and quickly became the fashionable method to perform internal bathing.

The medical staff at the spa at Plombières-les-Bains in France was one of the early and vigorous champions of internal irrigation. The full course of cleansing typically lasted from four to six weeks, with the treatment repeated every other day, or three times each week. The Plombières Douche became extremely popular, at least among the medical professionals prescribing it for their patients, and the procedure, or some close variant, was quickly adopted and administered in almost every spa in Europe and America that offered medical treatment.

The treatment was particularly popular at the spa at Harrogate, in northern England, where records show that 15,000 patients a year underwent the procedure.[34] Physicians reportedly administered 127,475 treatments between 1915 and 1925.[35] Physicians throughout England prescribed the "Harrogate cure" for patients who could afford it, and many insisted that it was the best way to treat their patients' ailments. Until about 1915 any medical skepticism about the effectiveness of the treatment was outweighed by the enthusiasm of the many physicians who believed that this was the only way for their patients to overcome autointoxication.

Colonic irrigation became the fad of the times, prescribed by a variety of practitioners from legitimate physicians who believed in autointoxication and wanted to cleanse the system without drugs, to unscrupulous quacks and hucksters who saw a demand and rushed to perform a service. As opposed to an enema, which typically cleared out only the rectum and part of the descending colon, an irrigation repeatedly rinsed the entire colon with large volumes of liquid. The concept was basically the same, to flush out the colon, but irrigation employed more elaborate equipment and did not lend itself to self-treatment.

An entire industry grew up to develop more and more exotic equipment to perform the task. Writing in 1914, physician Alcinous Jamison said, "Of late years inventive powers have been taxed to construct more convenient and effective appliances … [for cleansing the bowel]."[36] Many different models of irrigation apparatus appeared on the market, some of them extremely elaborate. Each designer felt that his complex apparatus was the best, and most incorporated water reservoirs, check-valves, water-level gauges, temperature controls, mixing valves, heaters, temperature gauges, inlet and output pipes, attachments for flushing away waste, and various complicated tubes for application. Equipment had impressive-sounding names such as "Suda-bad sub-aqueous colonic irrigator," first known as the "Enterocleaner" designed by Dr. Brosch of Vienna.[37]

While receiving treatment with the Gymnacolon Apparatus, developed by physician August von Borosini, the patient sat in a chair connected to a rotating frame that was then tilted so far back for treatment that the patient was horizontal with his legs stuck out in the air.[38] One competing design allowed the patient to be tilted even further until the individual was lying with their head downhill. The Studa Chair Apparatus did not tilt, but could be reclined almost like a bed.[39] Others exotic designs were the Dierker, the Vattenborg, the Schellberg, the Honsaker Lavagatory, and the Springfield.[40] The Dierker apparatus incorporated a vacuum system so that an internal intestinal massage could be administered at the same time as the irrigation by alternately expanding the colon with the pressure of gravity and then contracting it by means of a mild vacuum, thus alternately slightly blowing the patient's insides up and then deflating them back to normal.

One of the most elaborate piece of lavage equipment was the Subaqueous Intestinal Bath Apparatus. The patient reclined up to the neck in a bathtub full of warm water while receiving a continuous irrigation of the bowel through a complex series of rubber tubes and associated plumbing. This elaborate set-up included an underwater jet to provide massage of the abdomen to prevent cramping.[41] By 1922, approximately 10,000 colonic lavage treatments had been given in Vienna by the Subaqueous Intestinal Bath method. The clinic at Tübingen in southwest

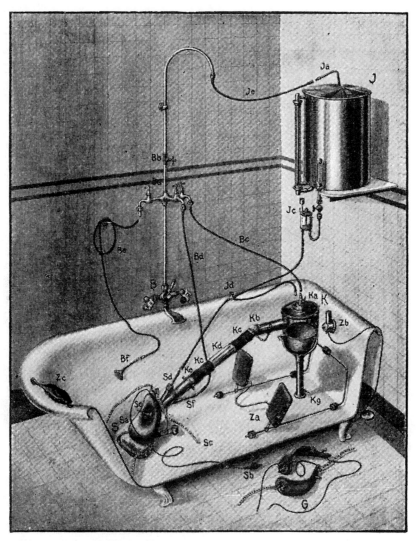

Fig. 16.—The Subaqueous Intestinal Bath Apparatus.

More and more complex devices for internal bathing were developed by eager physicians, each of whom thought he had developed the ultimate machine for the purpose. Probably the most complicated of these devices was the Subaqueous Intestinal Bath Apparatus. This complex explanatory diagram shows that treatment involved an intricate arrangement of interconnecting pipes, valves, and tubing, while the patient being treated was reclined submerged to the neck in a full bathtub while being simultaneously bathed by an underwater jet of warm water (Russell, *Colonic Irrigation*, 69).

Germany reported administering 12,430 of these treatments between 1922 and 1927.[42]

Some physicians felt that the use of all these elaborate machines, along with the rituals surrounding the preparation and treatment itself, made the patient feel that something positive was being done to help them, and may have indeed helped them, through the placebo effect.[43] This therapy was a relatively harmless practice and procedure that may have made the patient feel like they were gaining some benefit from it.

Physician William Kerr Russell, who specialized in colonic irrigation treatments in his practice, pointed out in the 1930s that lavage treatments administered with complex scientific-looking equipment by physicians or nurses dressed in formal white medical uniforms may have contributed to the placebo effect. Russell claimed that his patients reported that the treatment produced a feeling of well-being. He noted, "The treatment is also calculated to create the impression in the patient's mind that it will have curative action on his, or her, case…."[44] Russell often reported an increased appetite after the treatment, which gave more support to his theory that positive action in the form of this mildly invasive treatment made his patients feel better. Physician Alexander Gibson, who also made extensive use of irrigation, added, "Sometimes [afterwards] there is a sense of comfort, in which case we may presume that the lavage has done good."[45]

Charles Tyrell and Internal Bathing

In the early 1900s the popularity of bathing the outside of the body increased as the germ theory took hold and people realized that dirt contained bacteria that could lead to disease. As a result there was an increase in the advertising and sales of hand and body soap to promote cleanliness.

This time period coincided with a large growth in patent medicine sales. Laxative medicine manufacturers, in particular, quickly jumped on the bandwagon to promote internal cleanliness to remove "accumulated dirt" in order to promote better health. As one of the benefits of their products, patent medicine manufacturers commonly promoted extravagant claims for purification of the blood to remove the toxic byproducts of autointoxication by removing the bowel contents before they poisoned the body.

Others approached the market in a different way. Charles Alfred Tyrrell was a businessman who capitalized on and profited from the fears of autointoxication. Tyrrell later graduated from the Eclectic Medical College of New York in 1900, though he was already using the title of M.D. and usually also called himself "Professor" Tyrrell.[46]

One of the characteristics of a charlatan was to create a public persona for the masses by creating a suitably-impressive image of superior knowledge. Quacks took medical theories that had some degree of scientific basis, or at least a reasonable-sounding rationale, and inflated and molded this small bit of knowledge into a comprehensive explanation of the ailment they proposed to cure. They supported their claims with selected quotes from medical authorities and manipulated obscure medical statements into language suitable for the layman, making them sound like common sense.

Tyrrell's line of questionable reasoning that he put in front of the public started with two facts. Medical science had discovered that germs and bacteria cause disease, and the colon was full of bacteria. Then he drifted into the unsupported theory that illness was created in the large intestine by autointoxication and the toxic byproducts of these bacteria. The next step in his faulty chain of reasoning, the one where he overlaid his ideas on the scientific facts, was that to maintain health, these toxic byproducts should be washed out.

Tyrrell's print advertising describing the horrifying results of autointoxication was designed to create a morbid fear in the public that carrying around a load of toxic byproducts inside the body would create a dire threat to life itself. Then just when the reader despaired for his future health, Tyrrell stepped to the rescue with his answer that would alleviate the problem.

Tyrrell's advertising demonstrated the classic problem-solution approach of quack medicine. First, he created the dreadful problem in the minds of readers that autointoxication was bad and could cause grievous bodily harm. Second, he translated this into the desperate need for a product without which people could not live or the problem would become worse. Third, he provided the solution to the problem, namely that Professor Tyrrell just happened to have invented a device called the J.B.L. Cascade that would supply the perfect answer for the problem.[47] The J.B.L. simply stood for Joy, Beauty, Life. As Tyrrell explained it, "Without health there is no joy in life, and perfect beauty cannot possibly exist, while with health life becomes indeed worth living."[48] In the manner of the classic quack medical device, this type of science and reasoning had a dubious basis, and was then followed with an unproven non-sequitur, even though the logic sounded reasonable.

Tyrrell promoted internal bathing with his J.B.L. Cascade as the modern way to attain a youthful complexion, cleanse the skin, and achieve radiant beauty, and thus he and his ideas became part of the autointoxication lore. Washing out the digestive tract by giving it a Tyrrell internal bath became the new version of inner purification.

Tyrrell's convenient apparatus for internal bathing consisted of a five-quart rubber reservoir shaped like a hot water bottle, with a nozzle and stopcock on the upper surface. The user simply sat on the nozzle to insert it into the rectum, opened the valve, and the contents of the rubber bag were forced up into the colon by the user's weight, thus effectively flushing out all the toxic bacteria. In other words Tyrrell was simply selling a particular design of enema syringe.

In the flamboyant advertising style of the true charlatan, Tyrrell claimed that using his device "will give firmness to the tissues, elasticity to the step, color to the cheek, and sparkle to the eye." Then echoing the claims of the huckster, Tyrrell said that use of the Cascade "will positively CURE ANY DISEASE," except one, and even that is "not absolutely beyond hope." The implication was that the lack of a cure was not the fault of use of the Cascade, but that the patient was to blame. His advertising claims included a cure for appendicitis, dysmenorrhea, obesity, hemorrhoids, typhoid fever, scarlet fever, malaria, paralysis, and arthritis. Like many patent medicine hucksters, he used testimonials from satisfied customers in his advertising, at least from those who were favorably impressed with the product.

Tyrrell also played on the other everyday fears of many people. Tyrrell was quick to use everyday vague complaints and transient discomforts that most people occasionally suffered, such as irritability, depression, back pain, tender joints, headaches, shortness of breath after exertion, and an inability to move the bowels every day, as sure signs of autointoxication and the immediate need to use his device. For

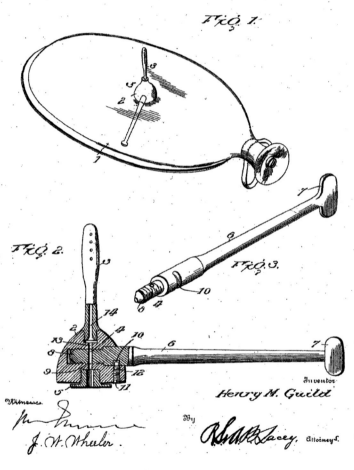

No. 757,654.

PATENTED APR. 19, 1904.

H. M. GUILD.

SYRINGE.

APPLICATION FILED AUG. 12, 1903.

MODEL.

FIG. 1.

FIG. 2.

FIG. 3.

Inventor

Henry M. Guild

Witnesses

J. W. Wheeler.

By

Attorneys.

In the early 1900s "Professor" Charles Tyrrell capitalized on the contemporary fears of autointoxication by promoting the J.B.L. Cascade, a device for flushing out the colon by sitting on a rubber cushion. Tyrrell developed an entire company and sales pitch devoted to the device and its accessories. With classic quack salesmanship, Tyrrell's advertising created a morbid fear of a nebulous condition, then offered a solution to the problem for a price. Sales of the Cascade continued to be strong into the 1940s (U.S. Patent Office, No. 757, 654).

example he claimed that young women who used the device regularly would have an improved complexion and figure that would make them attractive to young men, thus playing on the Victorian fears of sexual unattractiveness and spinsterhood.[49]

Another indicator of charlatanism is that Tyrrell created a variety of products to supplement the Cascade. One was Tyrrell's celebrated J.B.L. Antiseptic Tonic to be used with the Cascade device instead of plain water, to kill germs in the colon during the irrigation. In a different form, this was the old razor/razor-blade theory of advertising. In other words, sell them a razor that uses disposable blades and you will be creating a continued need to buy razor blades forever. In some cases it was even profitable to give away the razor, as the real profit came from constantly selling the razor blades. Tyrrell's antiseptic was advertised as the most perfect antiseptic in existence, along with being an internal healing tonic and muscle toner. Tyrrell sold his antiseptic powder for $1 for a one pound can, or $1.20 including postage if ordered through the mail. The American Medical Association estimated the manufacturing cost to be about five cents, thus leaving a hefty profit for Tyrrell.

Like many patent medicines, the exact composition of Tyrrell's powder remained a secret, which was also part of a marketing ploy that was supposed to indicate to the purchaser that it must be a very effective product if the formula had to be kept secret. After the passage of the Pure Food and Drug Act, the label on the can listed the ingredients as sodium bicarbonate, sodium chloride, menthol, eucalyptol, thymol, and borax. Basically it consisted of common table salt.

Similar to patent medicines of the time, the Cascade was promoted heavily through drug stores by using large window displays and advertising booklets titled "Why We Should Bathe Internally" for distribution to customers. The company engaged in mail-order campaigns with their booklet, follow-up mailings, and special offers to purchase the device. Tyrrell also published a thick book titled *The Royal Road to Health*, supposedly a medical text but in fact a thinly-disguised advertising for his product. The book was in print from at least 1899 to the 1920s. The 1917 version was listed as the 170th edition, and the book went into more than 260 editions.

The American Medical Association characterized the J.B.L. Cascade as "deceit, misrepresentation and quackery." Their opinion was that the use of the device was unscientific and could be dangerous in some cases.[50] But the public was reading newspapers and magazines, and listening to radio advertising that claimed that autointoxication was real, and that internal bathing was the most direct and natural method of keeping the bowels clean. What appeared contradictory to the public was that reputable physicians and sanitariums were irrigating patients' bowels in the name of autointoxication and medical science, but individuals were being told not to do the same for themselves at home.

Through clever and widespread advertising Tyrrell sold a large quantity of these devices. The price was $10 in 1900, which increased to $12 in the 1920s. The price was up to $12.50 in 1930. The Cascade was sold through the 1940s.

As usual, with the perceived popularity of the Cascade (in other words the large quantity of profitable sales noted by other eager salesmen), similar devices quickly came onto the market. By 1920, a wide variety of devices for internal bathing at home were available. Examples were the Davol Self-Administering Internal Bath, Hunt's Internal Bath, the Eager Internal Bath Appliance (from Eager Colon Cleanser Co.), and the Dupell Internal Bath.

The Jamison Internal Fountain Bath, designed by Alcinous Burton Jamison, a gastroenterologist from New York City who was another proponent of the theory of autointoxication, was never promoted as successfully as Tyrrell's product as it did not have the advantage of Tyrrell's doom-and-gloom advertising. The design was similar, but used a five-quart rubber bag shaped like a horseshoe, so that it could be placed directly on the toilet seat instead of on the lid, thus claiming more convenience for the user.[51] Jamison's device claimed double duty as it was also recommended for use as a hot water bottle, foot warmer, pillow, and invalid seat.

Jamison was a prolific writer who authored his own book titled *Intestinal Ills* and wrote an advertising brochure for Eager Colon Cleanser Company, which issued a brochure titled "Dr. A.B. Jamison's Fourteen Reasons 'Why the Internal Bath.'" In one of his books, Jamison recommended the use of his Internal Fountain Bath twice a day.[52] By 1914 and a new book he was recommending its use three times a day.[53]

Leaving aside for a moment the question of the dubious nature of this "treatment," Jamison is a good example of the blurring of the lines between the use and promotion of a product by a medical professional and a quack promotion of the same item. Jamison was a qualified physician and a leading gastroenterologist who promoted his own product. Tyrrell, on the other hand, had been labeled a quack by the AMA. He had self-bestowed credentials, opened his own "institute," and used the quack techniques of scary advertising and promotion for his product. But Tyrrell was the successful one.

The golden age of autointoxication lasted from about 1900 to 1930. Even by 1920 autointoxication as a useful diagnosis was falling out of favor among the medical profession. And even if kinks in the colon did cause stasis, which was still unproven, there was no evidence that this led to toxemia. Nobody had been able to show that any of these theoretically-toxic products were passed into the bloodstream. Though feces contained approximately 50 percent bacteria, it was never proved that any substances were being absorbed from the colon, and even if they were that they caused any illness or harm in the body.

By 1930 the medical profession had essentially abandoned the idea of autointoxication. Even so, the concept persisted among the general public. In the early decades of the 1900s, entire Victorian spas and clinics were centered around colonic irrigation. In the mind of the public this legitimized the treatment and the question in many minds was why not do it at home for a lot less money. An enema at home was cheaper and easier, as well as being a natural and painless way of clearing out the intestinal tract. A large quantity of enema equipment was sold in the 1920s because of the fears of autointoxication and the search for a simple, low-cost method of clearing the bowels of putrefying waste. Enemas were successfully promoted as an alternative to the unpleasant cathartics and unpredictable laxative patent medicines that were being advertised as cure-alls during the early 1900s.[54]

The large mail-order houses, such as Sears, Roebuck and Montgomery Ward, often devoted several full pages in their catalogs to advertisements for different syringes, euphemistically called "rubber goods," for flushing the insides cheaper and easier at home than paying someone else to do it. The 1927 Sears, Roebuck catalog, for example, contained twelve different models of syringe, including their house-brand version of Tyrrell's device.

This trend was also related to successful advertising campaigns of the 1920s that promoted popular worries in consumers about unpleasant bodily topics, such as various undesirable body odors, indigestion, constipation, bad breath, and other personal hygiene issues, linking them to the universal inherent desire to be beautiful and appealing. Creating and playing on consumer insecurities, advertising convinced potential customers that an important key to maintaining beauty, youth, energy, and attractiveness was to maintain a state of good health and personal purity. Advertisers promoted an obsession with cleanliness and good hygiene, attempting to make consumers believe that in this way they would become better, more attractive, and more desirable people. However, as an alternative viewpoint, some of the rise in sales of syringes for home hygiene may also be attributed to the increase in sexual experimentation during the 1920s flapper era. As author Therese Oneill has pointed out, the ideas of autointoxication and the need for internal cleanliness coincided with the rise of the use of douching for birth control before other methods were widely available.[55]

ELEVEN

Behold the Light

Visible light forms a narrow and specialized part of the total spectrum of radiant energy (see the appendix, *The Electromagnetic Spectrum*, for a very simple view of radiant energy). Light was significant to treatment of the body in two ways. One was treatment of the light receptors, the eyes themselves, which was often subject to the same odd variety of treatments as other parts of the body. The other was to use the radiant energy of different types of light as a method of treatment for various parts of the body.

Vision Treatments

In 1886 "Professor" William C. Wilson of Professor Wilson's New York & London Electrical Association of Kansas City (later the Actina Appliance Company) patented the Actina Eye Restorer for curing diseases of the eye. The device cost $10. Advertising by Wilson's company claimed that the device would cure all known diseases of the eye, including glaucoma, color blindness, and cataracts, which is a tall order even today.

The device consisted of a zinc cylinder that was chrome plated, about three inches long, shaped somewhat like a small trumpet, with a cup-shape at one end and a copper ribbon attached in a spiral to the outside. One end was for curing eye troubles and the other for the ear. Screw caps sealed the cylinder at each end. Electricity was supposedly generated when moisture from the skin came into contact with the combination of zinc and copper. It was touted as a "perfect galvanic and ozone battery."

Inside the cylinder was a piece of cotton cloth soaked in a mixture of oil of sassafras, mustard oil, belladonna extract, ether, and amyl nitrate. When the effectiveness of treatment appeared to be diminishing, the device could be "recharged" by sending it back to the company along with $1. Wilson re-soaked the muslin in his chemical mixture and returned it to the owner for reuse.

"Treatment" consisted of taking the end cap off the device and applying the cup shape to the closed eyelid and keeping it there for as long as the patient could tolerate it. Deafness and tinnitus (ringing in the ears) were treated by taking the cap off the other smaller end, inserting it into the nose, and breathing in deeply.

Associated advertising also promoted the same device as the Actina Pocket Battery, "a magic cure for headache, neuralgia, and colds in the head." More serious diseases, such as heart problems, cancer, and diabetes, were treated with the device in conjunction with special electromagnetic clothing that was conveniently sold by Professor Wilson.

Wilson sold 110,000 of the devices between 1885 and 1915. In 1915 the U.S. Postal Service finally issued a fraud order against the company, claiming that this was a scheme to fraudulently obtain money through the mail. This prevented the device from being sold through the mail and effectively stopped all sales.[1]

In the 1930s, another device for treating the eyes was the Natural Eye Normalizer, manufactured by the Natural Eyesight Institute. This chrome-plated metal device had two rubber eyecups designed to fit over the eyes, and a knob on the side. The user was instructed to place the device over the closed eyes and rotate the knob, an action that made the rubber eyecups move slightly and massage the eyelids. This questionable concept was supposed to relax the eyes and thus eliminate vision problems. Though the relationship to eye treatments seems somewhat tenuous, users were also advised by the manufacturer to sleep outside in the moonlight, to sunbathe in the nude between 11 a.m. and 2 p.m., and to walk in a bent posture on their hands and feet twice a week. Perhaps the only appropriate comment is that the owner of the Natural Eyesight Institute, Urbane Barrett, was convicted of mail fraud in 1937.

A similar mechanical device used for massaging the closed eyes was called the Neu-Vita Oculizer. It used a crank-and-pulley system to rotate the soft rubber eyecups. The device also had optional hard rubber eyecups that jabbed at the eyeballs when a rubber bulb was squeezed.

A device named the "Ideal Sight Restorer" was sold by Charles Tyrrell, manufacturer of the J.B.L. Cascade. The Restorer was supposed to correct all refractive errors of the eye, such as far-sightedness, near-sightedness, and astigmatism, as well as cataracts and glaucoma. The device consisted of two eyecups that were placed over the eyes, with an attached rubber bulb used to produce a partial vacuum over the eyeballs. The American Medical Association reviewed the device and determined that it was bogus.

Galvanic Spectacles

Galvanic Spectacles were an electrical invention from 1905 that had dark green lenses and a frame with electrical wiring in them that supposedly sent a stream of electricity to the optic nerve.

The glasses were invented in Connecticut in 1868 by Judah Moses, and a similar device was patented by John Leighton in England in 1888. These glasses had a chrome plate and a zinc plate in the frame that contacted the bridge of the nose when the spectacles were worn. A wire from each plate was attached to a small electric battery that supposedly delivered electricity to the bridge of the nose. This was claimed to stimulate the optic nerve. A supposed positive side effect was that use of the glasses was claimed to clear up sinus problems.[2]

Treatments with Sunlight

The concept of magical rays that supposedly promoted healing was an ideal concept for dubious treatments. The "magical" rays used for actual treatments included colored lights, infrared radiation, and violet ray generators.

Although many "light treatments" were completely without scientific foundation, the use of sunlight for the treatment of tuberculosis was a proven effective method. Two Swiss physicians, Bernhard and Rollier, were responsible for the medical acceptance of the usefulness of

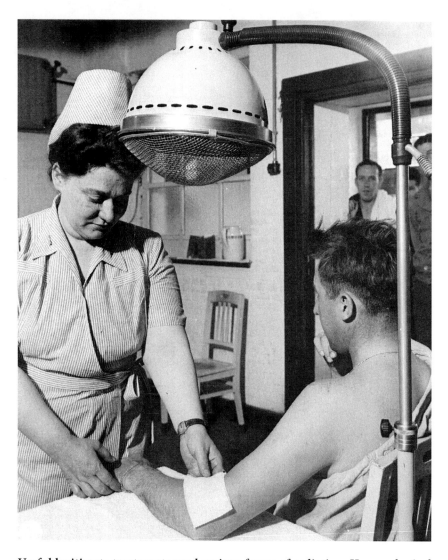

Useful legitimate treatments used various forms of radiation. Here a physical therapist treats the arm of patient, probably with either a heat lamp or with ultraviolet rays. Quack practitioners, on the other hand, used ordinary light-bulbs that were covered with theatrical filters to produce different colors of the visible spectrum that were supposed to cure various categories of illnesses (National Library of Medicine).

sun baths. The two practiced in the high alpine mountains of Europe, which had thinner air and where the sunlight was more powerful than at lower elevations. This was similar to towns in the western states in the United States that were tuberculosis treatment centers.

Tuberculosis, or TB for short, was widespread in the second half of the nineteenth century in America as a result of poor nutrition and crowded living conditions. The disease was more commonly known in Victorian times as "consumption" or as the "white plague." The reason it was called the "white plague" was that the disease caused the lungs to fill with white, spongy material. Eventually the victims suffered massive bleeding in the lungs and subsequent death. Because tuberculosis primarily affected the lungs, victims were known as "lungers."

The cause of tuberculosis was the bacillus *Mycobacterium tuberculosis*, which was spread by droplets from an infected person's cough. Consequently, the common practice of the time of spitting on sidewalks in public was a serious health problem. The bacterium was one of the oldest disease agents known to man and had probably been infecting humans for more than 10,000 years. The disease was primarily contracted by inhaling bacteria-laden air or by swallowing the bacterium in food or drink, particularly in milk from an infected cow. Direct contact, such as kissing, also transmitted the disease.

Until the true cause of the disease was discovered in 1882 by German bacteriologist Robert Koch, tuberculosis was thought to be cured by the intense sunlight and pure, fresh air of the mountains of the western United States. As a result, Colorado, Arizona, New Mexico, and California attracted many of those who had contracted the disease. Colorado was such a popular destination that it received the nickname the "World's Sanitarium." Indeed, "lungers" did seem to improve with the higher altitude and a regimen of outdoor living, eating healthy food, rest, fresh air, sunshine, and exercise. The improvement was probably due to these factors' boosting the victim's immune system, which helped to at least slow the worsening of the disease. Fresh air was an important part of the treatment and those with the disease slept in open, unheated, outside porches and lived in tent camps in all kinds of weather.

In 1902 Bernhard published the results of a study of the use of sunlight for sluggish wounds and external tuberculosis. In 1903 Rollier also started to use sun treatments for tuberculosis of the skin (lupus).[3] Exposure of various parts of the body to the sun for these treatments was called heliotherapy. One specific method was to use a mirror to reflect sunlight into the mouth and throat for treatment of tuberculosis in the throat. Although at one time heliotherapy was an accepted legitimate treatment, its application for the treatment of tuberculosis in no longer used, following improved methods of treatment with drugs.

A more dubious form of light treatment was the Radiant Ozone Generator that was patented in 1943.[4] The generator consisted of a wooden cabinet with a coiled glass tube, somewhat like those used in neon signs, on the top. The internal circuitry produced a high voltage to ionize gas in the tube that caused it to glow with red and blue colors. The device was advertised to treat arthritis, angina, diphtheria, whooping cough, kidney troubles, and many other ailments. In 1950 the FDA disagreed and declared the device misbranded.[5]

Infrared Radiation and Heat

Another way of treating the inside of the body was through the use of penetrating radiation. The "Burdick Infra-Red Generator" created radiation that was applied to the body by various means. The theory was that infrared rays penetrated the skin and provided heat to help blood flow in the tissues. Under his company name, Frederick Burdick himself wrote and published a 64-page book in 1923 that explained the rationale for the use of his machine. However, it was more of a tutorial on the physics of infrared radiation rather than a description of the actual conditions treated.

A chart at the back of the book listed pathological conditions where the use of infrared radiation, and specifically his device, would be beneficial. Among them were alcoholism, diabetes, appendicitis, gastric ulcer, gout, pancreatitis, and (in tune with the trends of the 1920s) auto-intoxication. A series of photographs and drawings showed the application of various Burdick devices for use with different external parts of the body, such as limbs and the trunk, and the attachments intended for internal body cavities.

Part of Burdick's rationale for using this infrared device was that heat had traditionally applied to the outside of the body to relieve pain, but that it only reached the outside of the skin and did not reach the internal parts. The Burdick generator solved this problem because the rays would provide penetrating heat that reached the internal organs via the use of a series of probes that were inserted into the vagina, bladder, and rectum.

The vaginal probe was used for treatment of "the various inflammatory, catarrhral and infectious conditions common to the female genitalia." The self-retaining rectal infrared dilator claimed "rectal dilation with Infra-red irridation [*sic*] relieves sympathetic tension and enhances portal circulation and elimination." The separate colonic applicator was long and slender and could be bent into any shape for higher insertion. The prostatic applicator, also inserted into the rectum, provided heat directly to the prostate gland via a special cup-shaped applicator.[6]

Another dubious electrical prostate treatment device was Vestvold's Improved Photo-Electric Dilator, developed by Rolf Vestvold in 1934. It was plugged into an electrical outlet through a cord at one end and into the patient on the other end, and delivered ultra-violet light to the colon to supposedly destroy the bacteria that caused autointoxication.[7] It was also recommended for use with diseases of the vagina.

Another device similar in concept for supplying heat internally for women was the Elliott thermophore, a legitimate medical treatment device for applying heat to a body part using heated water. In the Elliott device, a small rubber balloon was inserted into the vagina and supplied with water heated and circulated by a central control console. This supplied heat to the vagina, rectum, and adjacent internal tissues.[8]

Violet Ray Generators

Between 1830 and 1930, two radiation devices were heavily marketed to women, both supposedly used to combat the effects of fatigue and aging. One was the Electropoise described in Chapter Eight that was promoted to induce oxygen into the system. The other was the violet ray generator.

Violet ray generators were developed after electrical inventor Nikola Tesla in the United States and physician and physicist Jacques-Ansène d'Arsonval in France experimented with high-frequency alternating current. The violet ray device used a transformer to generate a very high voltage at a low current level that was then applied to a tube filled with a gas that glowed a deep purple color when it was stimulated by the electricity. When the applicator was held close to the body, it emitted sparks that jumped the gap to the skin. The violet ray was first demonstrated at the World's Columbian Exposition in 1893.[9]

Violet ray treatment machines came on the market in the early part of the twentieth century and were promoted to treat virtually every manner of ailment, including circulatory disorders, nervous affections, rheumatism, hair and skin disorders, sore throats, hemorrhoids, polio, female complaints, deafness, enlarged prostates, anemia, and catarrh.[10]

These violet ray machines, which generated a mysterious-looking violet glow with alleged therapeutic properties, were marketed by a number of manufacturers.[11] The violet ray generator was a handheld device. A handle with a glass applicator at the top radiated a stream of purple light that was supposed to treat the skin to enhance the appearance. Violet ray devices were also advertised to treat insomnia, headaches, weak lungs, hoarse voices, various aches and pains, and dandruff. One peculiar condition supposedly cured by the Master Violet Ray manufactured by the Master Electric Company in 1920 was a mysterious-sounding exotic ailment called "brain fog."

The Victorian era had different cultural ideals for men and women, thus medical devices were marketed differently to men and women, based on contemporary health and gender roles. For example, advertisements for electric belts showed sketches of muscular men with lightning bolts coming from them to imply men's bodies charged with powerful electrical forces. Electric belts were marketed primarily to men for strengthening virility, whereas violet rays and oxygen donors were marketed to women.

Men purchased electric belts and batteries for improving their manhood. Women, by contrast, purchased violet ray generators to improve their looks. Violet rays were supposed to ward off death and decay, factors that for women destroyed youth and beauty. Advertisements aimed at women emphasized the benefits of physical beauty. They showed the Electropoise and violet ray machines being used by women who were seductively posed lounging on a bed, as if being sexually charged by their devices. The women in these advertisements were portrayed as soft and beautiful. One advertisement for Roger's Violet Rays (1910) from Rogers Electric Labs showed a man's hand holding a wand massaging a woman's bare back. The implication was that use of the device produced desirable sexual attention by a man, and the hint that perhaps there was something further that he could do for her or with her.[12]

Violet ray machines emitted their brilliant, deep-purple ethereal glow via a variety of glass applicators. Applicators were specifically shaped for use on specialized places on the body or designed for insertion into various body orifices. Some models added vibratory capability and an ozone generator. Other attachments included steaming combs and facial massagers. The devices were particularly promoted to women for restoring youthful skin by stimulating circulation and eliminating cell waste in the blood.[13]

The term "violet-ray treatment" came to mean many different things and manufacturers started to make many extravagant claims. Some devices were high-frequency or high voltage, and some generated sparks. The common indicator was the violet color that appeared in the applicator.

The violet ray device produced by the Vi-Rex Electric Company in about 1900 was advertised for various treatments, though the conditions being treated were not always specifically or clearly spelled out, as the following shows. "The Violet Ray, as used in the treatment of the body, sends a spray of mild, tiny currents through every part and organ; flowing through each infinitesimal cell, massaging it, invigorating it, and vitalizing it." Potential customers were invited to send away for "A Book on Perfect Health via Vi-Rex Violet Rays—FREE."[14]

Shelton Laboratories sold sixty-three different electrodes for application to different parts of the body. Among them were electrodes with flat surfaces for general body treatments, one with a shape like a comb for pulling through the hair to treat dandruff and falling hair, a curved electrode for external use on the throat, a small cup-shaped electrode for use over the closed eye for weak eyes "to stimulate the optic nerves," a double eye electrode for treating both eyes at once, a tongue electrode for treating crevices in the mouth, and an ear electrode for treating "catarrhal deafness" and ringing in the ears. Metal electrodes were available for cauterizing, or searing the skin with caustic sparks. Urethral, rectal, and vaginal electrodes supplied with most generators were labeled as intended "for physician use," though their specific purpose and use never seemed to be really explained.

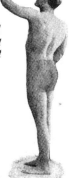
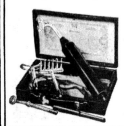
Violet ray generators, used to treat virtually every manner of ailment, were first demonstrated at the World's Columbian Exposition in 1893. The device used a transformer to generate a very high voltage that was then applied to a tube filled with a gas that glowed a deep purple color when it was stimulated by the electricity. These devices were particularly promoted to women for restoring youthful skin by stimulating circulation and eliminating cell waste in the blood (*Argosy All-Story Weekly*, Sept.1921).

The Renulife violet ray generator was made by Renulife Manufacturing Company of Detroit, Michigan, which sold a variety of models and electrodes. The Model E with one electrode sold for $24 in 1919. The fancier Model F, with a velvet-lined carrying case and two electrodes, sold for $30. The Deluxe Model C was supplied with the capability of providing different types of current for internal ("of exceptional smoothness") and external treatments, an ozone generator, and various electrodes, including a No. 16 eye electrode, a No 7 rectal electrode for prostate troubles, and a bottle of Renulife High Frequency Liniment. All for $75.[15]

Other devices were the Radiolux Violet Ray set (manufactured about 1930), the Shelton violet ray, and the Remco violet ray (the latter used for cauterizing small growths and moles using spark treatment). In 1920 the Lindstrom & Company of Chicago manufactured the Elko Electric Health Generator. The Elko Combination Health Generator No. 12 generated medical electricity, vibration, violet rays, and ozone all in one convenient device.

Violet ray generators reached the height of their popularity in the 1920s and 1930s. They were first promoted in the 1910s as cure-alls, but by the 1930s most of the device manufacturers were limiting their claims to skin treatment and beauty enhancement.

Violet ray devices were produced until the early 1950s, when the Food and Drug Administration halted their production. The remaining devices were turned over to the FDA in 1951 for destruction because they did not fulfill the promise of their benefits.

Colored Light Therapy

The use of colored visible light for healing was called chromotherapy. Two of the prominent systems were Spectro-Chrome light therapy and the Rainbow Lamp. Chromotherapy was also combined with radiesthesia, using a pendulum to indicate the correct color to use for subsequent therapy.[16]

Spectro-Chrome Therapy was invented by Col. Dinshah P. Ghadiali, who was born in Bombay, India, and moved to New Jersey in 1911. Ghadiali gave himself the title of M.D., though the American Medical

Association could find no record of this. He also claimed to be a doctor of chiropractic and doctor of philosophy. He said that by the age of eleven he was an assistant to a professor of mathematics at a Bombay college.

In 1920 Ghadiali invented the Spectro-Chrome Machine, which bathed the user in colored light, supposedly as a stimulant for the pituitary gland. The machine consisted of an elaborate box with an electric light in it that used various colored filters placed in front of the lamp to provide doses of colored light for treatment. He claimed that Spectro-Chrome therapy resulted in the "restoration of the human Radio-Active and Radio-Emanative Equilibrium by Attuned Color Waves." His slogan was "No Diagnosis, No Drugs.... No Surgery."

Ghadiali's concept was that the human body was composed primarily of oxygen, hydrogen, nitrogen, and carbon, which had the respective corresponding colors of blue, red, green, and yellow. In a healthy person, the four colors were equally balanced. When the colors were out of balance, disease was present. Thus, to cure disease and restore the balance, the practitioner administered the color that was lacking. The variations of colored light were also intended to treat a particular ailment or strengthen the body in a certain way. Red was supposed to be a liver energizer and hemoglobin builder. Blue was recommended as a vitality builder. Green light was a pituitary stimulant, a germicide, and a muscle tissue builder. Yellow light was claimed to be a digestant, an anthelmintic to expel intestinal worms, and a nerve builder.[17]

In the 1930s the smallest model of the Spectro-Chrome sold for $30. It consisted of a lamp housing with colored theatrical-gel filters placed in front of the light. A larger model used a 1,000-watt light bulb.[18] Glass or plastic slides were placed in a holder in front of the light in order to produce the colored light. The treatment consisted of the patient sitting fully unclothed in front of the Spectra-Chrome during the new moon or the full moon, while being bathed by different colored light. The light supposedly had to be applied to the bare skin as clothing would protect the patient from the treatment.

Ghadiali sold these devices for more than thirty-five years until he was prosecuted in 1945. He was found guilty when he went to trial because none of the colors were found to be effective for anything. In 1953 he founded the Visible Spectrum Institute and continued to sell his products. The lamps were labeled as having "no curative or therapeutic value" in order to avoid mislabeling charges, but amazingly they continued to sell. In 1958 a permanent injunction was issued against him and the sale of the Spectra-Chrome.

Others entrepreneurs developed similar devices. In Seattle in 1918 a homeopathic physician named Charles Wentworth Littlefield developed what he called a "Rainbow Lamp," that he used for treating almost every variety of ailment. He wrote a book titled *The Beginning and Way of Life* that was privately published in 1919, and had grandiose plans to build a Rainbow Temple in Seattle, with multiple rooms for light treatment.

William McKinley Estep invented a device called the Estemeter, though what it did and how it operated was obscure. It was apparently supposed to measure the acid level of the body, which was then used to determine an appropriate treatment plan with vitamins. The Food and Drug Administration confiscated a number of Estep's Roto-Rays, which consisted of a cabinet with a sun lamp, a short-wave unit, and colored slides. The concept was that the device was used to irradiate plain water which then became "atomic water" that was drunk to cure eighty-seven different ailments. As a result of FDA investigations, Estep was sentenced to three to five years in prison for medical malpractice.[19]

Light Baths

Being treated with light was not all totally bogus. One legitimate electric light bath that was used as a therapeutic device was popularized by John Harvey Kellogg at the Battle Creek Sanitarium. The technique involved putting the patient into a cabinet that was lined with electric light bulbs. Various combinations of these lamps were then activated to produce heat in the range of 110°F to 150°F. Similarly, the Greville Electric Hot Air Bath was used by doctors to treat one or two joints at a time, as the temperature could reach 300°F and its use was described as "somewhat trying."[20]

A more dubious electric bathing device was the MacGregor Rejuvenator from the 1930s. Its use was claimed to reverse the aging process and make people younger.

In 1932 William Mortrude of Seattle filed a patent on a device that was a large cylinder that looked like an iron lung from the 1940s or the more modern full-body MRI machine. The person being treated lay inside the cylinder, where he or she was bathed in AM radio signals, infrared light, and ultraviolet radiation.[21]

The Blue Glass Craze

One of the earliest light "cures" was the Blue Glass Craze of the 1870s. Supposedly a glass-making firm had made far more blue glass than they could sell. Trying to figure out what to do with it, one of the company's salesmen asked a friend who was a scientist if he could think of some new use for blue glass. The friend half-jokingly said that because the blue end of the visible light spectrum contained energy that acted on photographic plates, then this light should also stimulate tissues and cure disease. Intrigued by the concept, the salesman came up with the idea of advertising that claimed that blue glass was good for aches and pains. Surprisingly, the idea was well-received and the factory was able to sell its excess stock of blue glass. Furthermore, the popularity of the idea meant that they and other glass companies had to manufacture additional large quantities of blue glass to meet the new demand.[22]

One of those influenced by the concept was former Civil War General Augustus J. Pleasanton, who theorized that blue light was useful for the health of humans and helped to eradicate disease. He wrote a book titled *The Influence of the Blue Ray of the Sunlight and of the Blue Colour of the Sky: In developing animal and vegetable life; in arresting disease, and in restoring health in acute and chronic disorders to human and domestic animals,* in which he claimed that plants grown under blue glass flourished and pigs raised under blue grass put on more weight. This helped to further stimulate the "blue glass craze."[23]

As an extension of the blue glass concept, some doctors claimed that wearing blue-tinted eyeglasses would cure every ailment, so people started wearing tinted glasses. Some even replaced the windows in their houses with blue glass. Hotels replaced their clear plate-glass windows with blue glass, and streetcars in big cities installed blue glass in the windows of their horse-drawn carriages. Results, however, were reported to be mixed and people who had originally claimed a cure for their aches and pains went on to other "cures." Like other fads, the craze for blue glass faded away.

As an even more curious footnote to the blue light craze, recent observations in Japan seem to show that using blue lighting in railroad stations may lead to a decrease in the number of suicides from jumping in front of trains. In Nara, Japan, in 2005, and in Glasgow, Scotland, in 2000, the introduction of blue street lighting seemed to be possibly linked to a decrease in crime in neighborhoods that used these lights. Professor Tsuneo Suzuki, at Keio University in Japan, was of the opinion that blue lighting produced a calming effect in people; however, he also added that it was too early to draw any real conclusions.[24]

Whether it was just coincidental or not, blue was one of the colors widely used in Dinshah Ghadiali's Spectro-Chrome therapy. It was the color used initially to treat any condition of fever. Supposedly fever indicated an excess of hydrogen (red) and carbon (yellow) in the body, and using blue light produced the oxygen necessary for consuming the hydrogen and burning it into water. The result was supposed to be the perspiration that accompanied a fever. Oxygen also allegedly combined with the excess carbon and converted it into carbon dioxide which was harmlessly excreted from the body through the lungs and skin.

Twelve

The Promise
of Restored Youth

Anything to do with sex has always sold well, and many patent medicines and medical devices were sold in the Victorian era with the promise of restoring sexual vigor and vitality. Typical contemporary advertising gave hints of this with banner headlines such as "Private and Secret Diseases Particular to Men," referring in a subtle way to erectile dysfunction and sexually-transmitted diseases (STD). Particularly in the late nineteenth century and early twentieth century, quack medical device manufacturers created a fear through advertising that sexual weaknesses and diseases were rampant among American men. Those individuals with sexual issues were derisively called "weak men." Many people were embarrassed to approach their doctor about a sexual problem, but they could be persuaded by clever advertising to purchase a device or machine for self-treatment at home through the mail.

In the late 1800s new roles were forced on a society that had been recently industrialized with the technological advances that occurred after the American Civil War ended in 1865. Part of this change was a transition in traditional gender roles involving relationships between the sexes, and the interaction of the newly defined roles, physical functions, and behavior of men and women. Men and women had to redefine their roles in this new society. This was a male-dominated culture where men were supposed to support their families by working, and women's life was supposed to be a happy domestic mix of home and children. Part of the confusion of gender roles occurred because new opportunities were opening up for women with approaching emancipation. This rise in women's rights and changing attitudes towards sexual standards after the turn of the twentieth century contributed to male fears of inadequacy that sometimes became a self-fulfilling prophecy.

Part of the change in society involved who was responsible for moral behavior. In England until the 1750s, the Anglican Church had legal control over marital and sexual issues. After the Church lost its jurisdiction over sexual matters, it continued to influence people's marital and sexual practices, but it was essentially replaced by the medical establishment as the primary source of sexual control and advice.[1]

Physicians in both Britain and America increasingly took on the role of professional confidant and adviser for feelings, anxieties, emotions, and fears by administering to the sexual problems and fears of Victorian society. Patient confidentiality allowed a physician to share intimate secrets with the patient and take on a role of guidance in private family confidences. Because of this professional confidential relationship with a patient, doctors also started to take on the role of moral controller. They used their status as medical men to try to influence the community by dispensing their own opinions on sexual activity. In doing this, they found themselves facing all the problems of sexuality, which included the lesser allied categories of drug abuse, personal hygiene, marital relations, contraception, masturbation, and impotence.[2]

As one example, by the mid–1800s, physicians, health reformers, purity authors, and food faddists had made up a list of foods they felt should be forbidden, such as tea, coffee, chocolate, tobacco, and alcohol. These items, along with flesh meat, oysters, and eggs, were theorized to irritate the nervous system and inflame sexual desires, which reformers felt should not be allowed. Condiments, such as salt, pepper, mustard, cloves, ginger, and mace, and fine-flour breads, were unequivocally stated to inflame the nerves of the sexual organs and produce "morbid desires."

With an increasing role in sexual matters, many doctors convinced themselves that they were responsible for the morals of mankind and brought their professional scrutiny to focus on issues that they felt threatened the stability of contemporary society. Physicians even offered advice to women on beauty and general body hygiene. Some of their questionable advice included the proper sizes for breasts, including the measurements and dimensions, and the optimum size for a woman's neck and waist.

The history and study of Victorian sexuality is a complex and sometimes conflicting one. The medical profession and most males viewed it from a male androcentric viewpoint. Marriageable women were conceptualized as passionless and above carnal desire, and only participated in sex in the interests of matrimonial harmony and motherhood. The reality ranged from the opinion of physician William Acton, who solemnly pronounced that women had no sexual feelings at all, to that of contemporary women's diaries that revealed that some women found sex to be very enjoyable.

Men, on the other hand, were officially considered to be dominated by their carnal desires and needed sexual release periodically in order to stay healthy. This led to the double standard that was used to justify prostitution. There were two basic categories of women. Good women, who were for marrying, and the other kind to have fun with. Masturbation was problematic as the practice was considered to be unhealthy, but men were assumed to need periodic sexual release to maintain good health.[3]

Another factor was the emergence in the last part of the nineteenth century of the professional sexologists, who tried to make sexual behavior the subject of scientific study. Two of the leaders in the field were Sigmund Freud and British sexologist Havelock Ellis, who wrote the massive seven-volume *Studies in the Psychology of Sex* between 1898 and 1928.

Sexologists and physicians developed their own opinions of sexual behavior and felt that everyone should follow these ideals. Some of these ideas reached the ridiculous. For example, one was that the practice of dancing as a couple should be limited because a woman could absorb a male's domineering and passionate nature through magnetic contact while on the dance floor.

Along with the professionals came the quacks, in the form of unofficial medical practitioners who did a booming business in various cures for sexual ailments. They advertised and operated largely through the media of the day, which was newspapers, magazines, mail order advertising, and other print media. Another sales outlet for their wares was door-to-door salesmen, who concentrated on sales to urban class neighborhoods.

Impotence

Impotence was an absence of sexual power and a failure to achieve an erection. Mesopotamian medical texts as far back as the seventh century BC contained recommendations that men eat certain roots and plants to restore their potency. The word "impotence" came into the common vocabulary in the seventeenth century, though for centuries before that men had complained about a "loss of courage" and "lack of desire." And indeed the fear still exists among modern males.

The Victorian model of masculinity contained a strong cultural fear of male sexual inadequacy. Potency was importance for a man's reputation, and male impotence was a serious deficiency when family inheritance and financial fortunes depended on having children. Sexual virility was associated with youth, and an erection was physical proof that a male could lead life properly as a man.[4] The erect organ was a Victorian symbol of maturity, power, and manhood. For many men, sexual strength also represented social dominance over women, thus any failure in that area was perceived as weakness.

Today urologists blame impotence (now called erectile dysfunction) on poor blood circulation and can offer several medications to improve performance, but in previous times men resorted to other means. Quick to note a need to be filled, quacks employed advertising both to create personal anxieties in potential customers and to sell their own methods to cure "lost manhood."

The Male Drive to Be Young Again

At the turn of the twentieth century there was a steady growth of sex aids to treat "diseases of men" or "secret diseases." They were aimed primarily at men, mostly targeted towards the older male who wanted to retain or restore youthful vigor. Some were outright frauds, such as Vital Sparks, a medicine that was advertised to boost male virility. In reality, Vital Sparks consisted of pieces of hard black candy rolled in powdered aloes. The label on the small pasteboard package said that it was "God's Great Gift to MEN," the inference being obvious.

Many patent medicines claimed to resolve impotence. As early as

1739, Prolifick Elixir was guaranteed to "raise their inclination." Dr. Brodum's Nervous Cordial and Botanical Syrup offered "to make men ready for the married state." Samuel Solomon's Cordial Balm of Gilead (a mixture of cardamom, brandy, and cantharides) was recommended for curing impotence. James Hodson's Persian Restorative Drops guaranteed "to overcome a loss of firmness and vigor."[5]

Among other non-drug treatment methods were the use of hydrotherapy, electrotherapy, acupuncture, insertion of bougies and sounds into the urethra, and use of a vibrator.[6] Vigorous horseback riding was reportedly used as one nineteenth-century treatment for impotence.[7]

Treatment devices included penile splints, rings, and vacuum pumps, all intended to improve performance and restore the male ego. Among the splints was The Robut-Man, sold by Presto Products of Chicago, Illinois, a hard rubber device that came in various sizes, according to measurements supplied by the user. For cases where "nature fails entirely," the company recommended that the buyer "use the WONDER MONSTER AUTO-MAN, the mechanical penis." The company also sold two different types of vacuum pump for organ enlargement.

The Scientific Appliance patented by Professor Bartholomew in 1900 for the relief of impotence was manufactured in small, medium, and large sizes. It was advertised as "A Boon to Men" and "Nature's Cure for Loss of Manly Power Without Drugs."[8] Similar were Bier's Erectruss, another penile splint, and the Sklerator.[9]

The Sklerator was a celluloid cylinder placed around the penis and held to the body with a rubber band. It was intended to increase the flow of blood during initial erection. The inventors believed that the use of the device also had a psychological effect on potency and increased male self-confidence.[10]

One of the effective mechanical devices for maintaining and developing an erection worked by compressing the veins in the penis and preventing them from emptying too rapidly. A similar purpose was served by the Obturator, a device worn over the penis, invented by a Dr. Williams. Made of soft rubber, it compressed the blood vessels at the base of the penis to slow down the return flow of blood.

The Potentor, invented by Dr. Kratzenstein, was an inflatable ring that also created pressure on the return blood vessels and prevented deflation due to the return flow of blood. Advertising for the product claimed, "Shortly after wearing the Potentor one should experience a feeling of well-being, GREATER EASE OF ACTIVITY, bouyance [sic], cheerfulness, more joy and interest." Appealing to male wishes, the manufacturer promised, "The Potentor is designed to stimulate pep, vim, vigor and vitality, and corrects what has gone wrong." It was indeed "A New Road to 'Strongville.'"

Similar to the contraptions used to try to increase bust size in women were vacuum pump devices that were placed over the penis to increase blood flow to the organ. They typically promised to enhance size, like the breast enlargers intended for women.

All were essentially the same type of device. The basic principle was exemplified by the Vital Power Vacuum Massager, developed by W.J. Lynch of Springfield in 1921. The user placed a glass (later plastic) cylinder over his penis, held it tight so that a rubber gasket at the base formed a seal to the abdomen, and turned a hand-operated crank to create a vacuum inside the cylinder. According to one advertisement for the Vital Power Vacuum Massager from Bottlers Supply Company of Springfield, Illinois, this method caused a powerful suction action to draw blood into the penis, "causing normal, natural nourishment, resulting in A FLOW OF HEALTH, VITALITY and POWER, and complete development of abnormal and undersized parts." The pump was promoted in another full-page advertisement as the "Perfect Organ Developing Appliance. Invigorates, Enlarges Shrunken and Undeveloped Organs."[11]

A device invented by Carl C. Lanz from New York City also used an attached rotary handle on the end, which the user cranked to produce the vacuum. The one made by the Vital Gland Power Company used a bicycle pump to create a vacuum. In a clever stroke of marketing, this company used testimonials from older men in their eighties to promote the product, but their sales force consisted almost entirely of young women.[12]

Similar were the Vital-O Vacuum Developer, advertised as "A Remarkable Instrument for Underdeveloped Organs." It consisted of a glass tube, about eight inches long and an inch and three-quarter inches in diameter, that was attached to a vacuum pump. Vim Manufacturing's Juvenator had a glass container the end of which was attached to a "powerful nickel-finished vacuum pump." Fred Leach, under the name of the Vacuum System Company, made a "Vacuum Developer for Men" until the Post Office issued a fraud order against him.[13]

The Strenva Company sold a similar vacuum appliance "for the cure of diseases of and the development of the male sexual organs," until a fraud order was issued against the company in 1905 for false and fraudulent claims.[14]

The Springer Self-Treating Device developed in 1920 by W.T. Springer of Springer Treating Device Co., of Waterloo, Iowa, was far more complex. His device treated impotence with the combined use of hot water, an induction coil, an electric current, a vacuum, and an electrode that was inserted into the rectum for a "prostate massage," all at the same time.[15] Advertising promised "The Way to Health thru Enforced Circulation of the Blood." He claimed that it worked through "enforced hyperemia," which simply means to say that the device increased the flow of blood in that particular part of the body.

To operate the device, the patient's genitals were covered with a metal hood connected to a vacuum pump. One pole of a battery was connected to the metal hood, the other to the electrode inserted into the rectum. Then the vacuum pump was energized to create a vacuum, and the electric current was turned on and gradually increased. The combination of the stimulation of the electric current and the vacuum surrounding the penis was supposed to strengthen it. A corresponding model was available for women. Following other not untypical quack distribution schemes, part of their advertising noted, "exclusive territory given to doctors."

Once electrical treatments became fashionable, electricity and magnetism were soon claimed to cure loss of erectness. Galvanic cures were offered by both conventional physicians and quack doctors. One recommended treatment for impotence involved attaching a zinc-lined electrode in the shape of a cylinder around the penis or inserting an electrode into the urethra and delivering a strong jolt of electricity.[16]

The most popular impotence cure between 1890 and 1920 was the electric belt, which was described in detail in Chapter Eight. Available through mail-order, impotence remedies such as the electric belt allowed men to do something in secret about their condition without

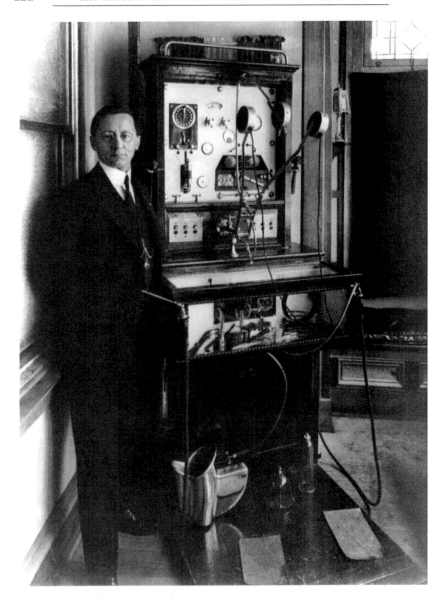

This is Dr. Richard R. Schleusner in 1921 standing next to his intriguing apparatus for "restoring youth to the aged." Looking very complex, with switches and rheostats mounted on the front panel and what appears to be glass suction devices on the floor in front of the machine, no further information seems to be available on what the device was supposed to accomplish or how it did it. This machine appears to have similarities to the Stringer [*sic*] Self-Treating Device pictured in McCoy (*Quack*, 213) and, given the cryptic description, may have served the same purpose (Library of Congress).

the embarrassment of going to see a doctor or shopping in a pharmacy. Men could treat impotence without even their wives knowing.

The electric belt companies also used the quack marketing man's technique of creating a fear and need in the customer, then selling him the solution to the problem. Belt companies advertised to men that impotence was caused by lost vital energy due to youthful masturbation and that use of their belt could restore this energy and replace the drain on vital forces. They intensified the Victorian fears of the result of masturbation as a youth by offering a list of vague symptoms that any man could be suffering from, such as tiredness, nervousness, bad moods, and frequent headaches. The list of ghastly consequences inferred that the youthful masturbator would end up in an asylum if he didn't buy their particular brand of electric belt in a hurry and start using it.[17] In this way the belt manufacturers provided a clear diagnosis of the problem and offered a product for purchase to effect a cure.

Typical electric belts were the Samson Electric Belt and the Sanden Electric Herculex No. 8 that were recommended for sending current through the body to combat cases of sexual weakness, nervous debility, and prostate troubles. Advertising pictures for the devices typically showed small lightning bolts radiating from the electric battery discs in order to imply the belt's power. Another advertising ploy was to show a discreet sideways picture of a naked man wearing the belt, with little lightning bolts radiating out from the hidden genital area of his body added to the picture.

Men became absolutely preoccupied with the issue and, by the 1890s, Victorian men were being subjected to a barrage of quasi-medical advice from both legitimate physicians and quack doctors. Even mesmerists claimed to be able to offer relief.[18] Many of the quack advertisements that appeared in the newspapers, and especially in the cheap press, exploited men's sexual anxieties. Typical were "lost manhood" advertisements offering all sorts of apparatus for restoring weak erections. This included advertisements for devices such as Dr. McLaughan's Electric Belt, which often appeared on the back page of the *National Police Gazette*, the crime and sporting tabloid that always had advertisements for men's "restoratives."

Boyd's Battery

In the nineteenth century, quack doctors claimed that the main cause of impotence was masturbation.[19] Frederick Hollick, the author of the long-winded *A Popular Treatise on Venereal Diseases, in All Their Forms. Embracing Their History, and Probable Origin; Their Consequences, Both to Individuals and to Society; and the Best Modes of Treating Them,* claimed that people who masturbated or suffered from nocturnal emissions would experience mental imbecility or "softening of the brain" and that any misuse of the sex organs put nasty little boys in danger of becoming insane.[20] Masturbation, also known as the "solitary vice," "self-abuse," and "self-pollution," was the ultimate Victorian taboo throughout the Victorian era and for a long time afterwards.[21] Moralists regarded the practice as sinful and psychologically damaging, and created inflated fears that it was medically dangerous and physically harmful.

One of the advertising pitches that addressed the solitary vice that Victorians dreaded so much included the ominous accusation: "Did you, when young, draw unnaturally on the fountain of life and strength, one drop of which fluid is equal to thirty drops of the heart's blood." In typical patent medicine advertising fashion, Professor Boyd had just created a dreadful health problem that all men feared. Then he offered the solution: "…there is no remedy that will relieve all the ailments caused from self-abuse with such magic as Boyd's Miniature Galvanic Battery." Thus Professor Boyd solved a serious problem in the privacy of the home for only a few dollars.

Boyd's Miniature Galvanic Battery, patented in 1878, consisted of a series of twelve small, pill-shaped discs made from different metals, then assembled together in a flat, disc-shaped housing with the ends of the metal pills exposed. Supposedly the different metals in contact with each other and the skin created a galvanic battery. The entire device was about the size and thickness of a fifty-cent coin. A silk cord was attached so that the battery could be worn around the neck. The battery was supposed to be worn day and night for at least a month after the patient was cured.

And there was one even more dubious claim. As Professor Boyd explained the theory, "the various blocks of metal were so placed that when the electricity was formed it would be formed in the gimlet shape, and he said it would enter the system in that form and pass on twisting until it spent its force."[22]

The rationale for the device was the classic synthesis of real science combined with a theory that extrapolated the explanation into bogus reasoning. Boyd quoted the scientific fact that English physician William Harvey had described the circulation of blood in the human body. This was a well-established fact that gave the rest of the pseudo-science an air of credibility. Boyd then went on to say that if the blood could be infused with electricity as it passed by the battery, the blood and nerves would be invigorated "with new electric life." He then followed with the common idea of the time that disease was caused by "impure blood." The next leap of faith for the consumer was that wearing Boyd's battery would cure a whole host of horrible-sounding ailments.

For an entire loss of manhood, Boyd recommended that two batteries be worn at the same time, one around the neck and one between the shoulder blades. Presumably in an effort to promote sales, he recommended that the same battery should not be worn by different people as this would transmit the disease from one to the other.

Richardson's Magneto Galvanic Battery, patented 1891, was much the same.

The Orgone Accumulator

In the 1940s, recharging a person's orgone energy level was thought to be the newest scientific method to restore "lost vitality" and invigorate the sex life.

The promoter of orgone energy was Dr. Wilhelm Reich. Reich was born in Austria in 1897. He received his M.D. degree from the University of Vienna Medical School in 1922 and studied under Sigmund Freud, who was working in the new field of psychoanalysis. Reich subsequently moved to Berlin, where his views became unpopular with the government, so he fled to Scandinavia and then moved to the United States in 1939. Reich held a number of teaching and administrative posts, including associate professor at the New School for Social Research in New York.

In 1938 Reich published a book titled *Die Bione: zur Entstehung des vegetativen Lebens*, which described his theory that the fundamental life force was the "bion," a microscopic, cyst-like sac filled with orgone energy, which was a rudimentary form of life developed from inorganic matter. Reich claimed that orgone was a form of non-electromagnetic life force energy that permeated all of nature. It was in the soil and the atmosphere, and in all plants and animals. It reached earth from outer space, but was not detectable by conventional scientific instrumentation (like many forms of healing energy associated with quack devices).

Reich theorized that orgone in the human body was the basis of sexual energy or, in other words, that it was orgasmic energy. He claimed that the erogenous zones of the body were infused with orgone energy during the sex act, that it was the energy released during orgasm, and that it had natural healing powers.[23]

Reich felt that orgone arriving on earth was related to static electricity and explained heat waves, the blue color of the sky and oceans, thunder clouds, lightning, radio interference, and many other natural phenomena. He further theorized that many diseases were the result of insufficient or restricted orgone flow.[24]

In 1940 Reich invented the Orgone Energy Accumulator to absorb and store this mysterious energy. The accumulator was a large, empty wooden box, spacious enough to sit in, measuring approximately five feet high, two feet wide, and two-and-a-half feet deep, lined with sheet iron on the inside and wood on the outside. The door was lined with sheet iron. Later versions were made from alternating layers of steel wool and rock wool. The multiple-layer construction was supposed to concentrate even higher levels of energy.

The theory was that orgone energy was attracted by the wood layer on the outside of the box, passed through the metal layer, and radiated into the inside of the box. The metal contained and reflected the energy once it was inside, and thus was able to build up a high concentration of energy in the box.

The patient being treated sat inside the box on a chair for ten to thirty minutes at a time, wearing light clothing (or better yet no clothes at all) to charge up their body with orgone energy, which would supposedly improve their health. Supposedly patients would eventually feel a warming sensation, which was a sign to stop the treatment before

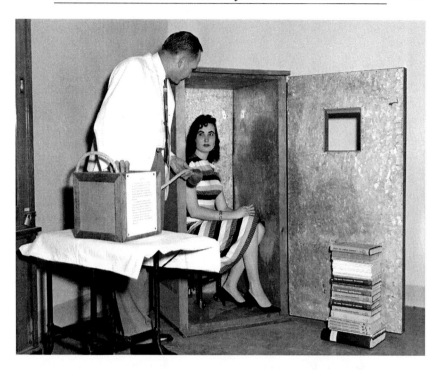

In the 1940s, recharging a person's orgone energy level by sitting inside an Orgone Accumulator was thought to be the newest scientific method to restore "lost vitality" and invigorate the sex life. Designed by Dr. Wilhelm Reich, the Accumulator was a large wooden box lined with sheet iron on the inside and wood on the outside, with a door lined with sheet iron. The box was intended to contain and reflect orgone energy inside, and build up a high concentration of this nebulous energy in the enclosure. The stack of books holding the door open are all publications by Reich. The tin funnel the practitioner is holding is attached to an associated breathing apparatus in the box on the table (U.S. Food and Drug Administration: FDA 138).

nausea or dizziness occurred. Reich claimed that the box eventually glowed with all this energy.

Reich presumed that his invention could cure almost any disease, and he told patients that even life-threatening diseases could be treated by sitting in the Orgone Energy Accumulator. For example, this mysterious orgone energy could cure colds, arthritis, anemia, ulcers, and skin abrasions. Among other beneficial effects, Reich felt it was also helpful for treating fatigue, migraine, chronic colds, early stage cancer, arthritis, sinusitis, and any type of wound. In fact, it supposedly sterilized wounds. One of the stranger claims was that Reich's discovery could be used to immobilize bacteria in the vagina by inserting a glass pipe filled with steel wool.[25] Reich developed a special version of the Accumulator for bed-ridden patients, which consisted of layers of material that were placed underneath and on top of the patient.

Reich also used the Accumulator to treat a multitude of psychological problems and character traits that he felt were undesirable, some of which were related to sex. The final goal of the psychological part of the therapy was the treatment of neuroses and developing the patient's ability to have a full and complete orgasm. He had his patients sit in the Accumulator to build up their orgone levels (i.e., sexual energy) and build up the libido. Obviously some practitioners believed in Reich and his methods, as the Food and Drug Administration estimated that he sold more than a thousand of the Accumulators.

Reich founded the Orgone Institute in Forest Hills, New Jersey, but eventually it was shut down by the FDA. He also developed a device called a Cloudbuster that had large fifteen-foot hollow aluminum pipes that were pointed at the sky to pull down orgone energy. After some controversy arose about his theories and methods, Reich exhibited some of the signs of quackery discussed in Chapter Two, and started to speak out about an international conspiracy to suppress knowledge about orgone. About the same time he also claimed that extraterrestrial beings were threatening the earth.[26]

Scientists at the FDA concluded that there was no such energy as orgone and that the Accumulators were worthless for the treatment of disease. In 1954 the FDA ordered Reich to stop shipping Orgone Energy Accumulators and filed an injunction against the interstate shipment of the devices. Reich continued to ship Accumulators and was brought to trial in 1956. He was found guilty of contempt of court and sentenced to two years in prison. Reich went to federal prison and died there in 1957.[27]

James Graham and the Celestial Bed

James Graham was a Scotsman from Edinburgh who has been given the dubious title of the "Emperor of Quacks." Graham studied medicine at Edinburgh University and was an enthusiast of medical electricity. He practiced in England in Bristol in 1774, then in Bath, using electrical cures. In one part of his therapy he placed patients on magnetic chairs. Mud baths were high on his list of treatments for long life and sexual rejuvenation, though his personal supervision of mud baths involving nude women perhaps made that part of his medical motives somewhat suspect.[28]

In 1780 Graham opened an establishment in London that he named the Temple of Health. Customers could obtain Graham's medicines, such as "Electrical Ether," "Nervous Ethereal Balsam," and "Imperial Pills," while breathing "electrical, dephlogisticated and vivifying atmosphere."[29] Graham supposedly treated 200 patients a day.

For £2 an interested visitor could hear a lecture about health, sex, and beauty, given by "Doctor" Graham himself, assisted by scantily-clad "goddesses of health."[30] He also titled himself "John Graham, O.W.L." The initials stood for "Oh Wonderful Love."[31] This type of egotistical affectation was similar to the E.R.A. (Electronic Reactions of Abrams) of Albert Abrams, the J.B.L. (Joy, Beauty, Life) Cascade of Charles Tyrrell, and the more egotistical I-ON-A-CO of Gaylord Wilshire.

Graham's specialty was fertility. For a suitable fee, patients could sleep overnight in his Celestial Bed to "awaken the dormant generative powers" of a couple and improve their sex life. He claimed that its use would overcome sterility and impotence. The goal was to induce conception for those couples who desired children.[32]

The Celestial Bed was large in size, twelve feet long and nine feet wide, supported by forty glass pillars, and covered by a dome with the figures of Cupid and Psyche on the top. The inner frame of the bed could be inclined at different angles to supposedly assist in conception. The mattress was stuffed with stallions' tails and mirrors lined one side. To provide suitable encouragement for those using the bed, at the head was the motto, "Be fruitful, multiply and replenish the earth." During use, exotic perfumes wafted around through the air, soft music played, incense burned, and colored lights glowed. Graham's cost for this setup was estimated at £10,000.

Graham claimed that the bed operated by magnetism and electrical fire. Underneath the bed, 1680 pounds of magnets, which gave it the name of "Celestial or Magnetico-electrico Bed," supplied magnetic power to ensure fertility. The Celestial Bed was surrounded by costly draperies and stood on glass legs to insulate the magnetic currents from the ground. Graham called the mechanism "magneto-electrical healing," but did not have any scientific proof for its operation, or even a scientific reason, but he had a good sales pitch. Graham promised that those wishing to conceive could spend a night on the bed for £50 and enjoy "superior ecstasy" "accompanied by soft music."[33]

Graham obviously had some insight into the psychology of impotence, and was aware of the influence of fantasy and imagination in sexual performance. He counted on the likelihood that use of the Celestial Bed would stimulate libido and desire through ambience and expectation, with the accompaniment of soft music, perfumes, and lighting. Some of the couples using his bed indeed may have had psychosomatic failings and just needed the encouragement provided by stage props and a romantic atmosphere, coupled with Graham's reassurance that the bed would work. The Celestial Bed initially received immense popular interest, but enthusiasm for its use had waned by 1783.

Gland Transplants

Impotence and the male failings that come with age have always been a subject of great interest and concern for men.

Dr. Serge Voronoff, an eminent Russian-born surgeon practicing in France and Egypt, claimed that the aging process and subsequent decline in sexual capability for men was due to a decrease in hormonal activity. He theorized that the sex glands wore out and resulted in aging, so his idea was to give the older body a boost by implanting the testicles of young animals into old men. He felt that in this way the aging process could be reversed.[34]

In 1917 Voronoff started animal experiments in Paris and in 1920 started to implant small amounts of monkey testicles into patients. He reasoned that the small slivers he used would be absorbed into the system and rejuvenate the patient's sex life. Voronoff even lectured on the subject to the International Congress of Surgeons in London in 1923, claiming that the results of the transplant were increased sex drive, increased energy, better eyesight, and longer life. The cost of his surgery was $5,000.[35] About the same time, Dr. Egen Steinach of Vienna was doing the same.[36]

A similar solution for impotence was marketed in the 1920s and 1930s in the United States by Dr. John Romulus Brinkley. Brinkley had three medical degrees, two of which were from bogus medical diploma mills, the Bennett Medical College of Chicago and the Eclectic Medical University of Kansas City.[37]

In August of 1918, Brinkley opened a sixteen-room clinic in Milford, Kansas, called the Brinkley Institute of Health. Here he implanted small pieces of goat testicle into the scrotums of male patients to allegedly improve their virility. During the 1920s Brinkley performed these goat gland operations on thousands of patients. The basic fee for the gland surgery was $750, increasing to $1,500 for using a very young goat.

The concept of becoming younger through gland implantation was used by Arthur Conan Doyle in a Sherlock Holmes short story titled "The Adventure of the Creeping Man," published in 1923. In the story, Professor Presbury, an older man of sixty-one, intends to marry a much younger woman and wishes to rejuvenate himself and regain some of his youthful powers. To achieve this he gives himself a series of injections with a serum made of extracts from a climbing monkey. The unfortunate result is that Presbury himself is transformed periodically into the same type of climbing monkey.

Stimulating Glands the Hard Way

Men have always been concerned with virility, and manufacturers stepped forward with quack devices that were advertised to assist with overcoming impotence and other sexual problems. The concept of stimulating the glands to restore sexual performance by doctors like Voronoff and Brinkley was immediately noted and acted upon by the manufacturers of unusual medical devices. Several manufacturers made devices to go right to the alleged source of the trouble, the male prostate.

At the time, on-going legitimate scientific medical investigation stimulated new interest by the public in the human glands. Quacks immediately jumped onto the bandwagon and combined this legitimate research with pseudo-scientific information. They convinced men in particular that proper functioning and control of the glands, particularly the prostate, was the key to physical, personal, and sexual success. They promised that use of their products would produce an unlimited sex drive and eternal life.[38] The implication was that neglected glands would be unhealthy and lead to sexual dysfunction.

To provide treatment to this particular internal part of the body, the manufacturers of quack medical devices needed some convenient way to access the inside of the lower part of the abdomen, in particular the prostate, to apply an internal treatment directly to the gland itself. The only reasonable way to reach the prostate other than surgery, which was obviously not feasible, was by inserting devices into the nearest natural body orifice, in this case the rectum. Indeed, this is still the legitimate route for performing examinations of the prostate.

One way advertised to achieve treatments was with Dr. Young's Ideal Self-retaining Rectal Dilators, a set of four devices of increasing sizes. They were made from hard rubber, and increased in size from a half-inch to one inch in diameter, and from two inches to four inches in length. The cost was $3.75 for the set of four. For use, one of the devices was inserted into the rectum for treatment of chronic constipation and hemorrhoids. The method was also claimed to treat "dyspepsia, rheumatism, insomnia, asthma, disease caused by sluggish circulation, and malnutrition."[39] For men, they were particularly recommended for "prostate troubles." Without saying exactly how or why they were supposed to produce their healing magic, their use was also claimed to be "wonderfully beneficial" for women during pregnancy and menstruation. Young's Dilators were sold from the late 1800s until 1940, when they were seized and charged by the Food and Drug Administration as being mislabeled.

Similar devices were Kelly's Dilator and Pratt's Dilator, which were used to stretch a tightly contracted sphincter due to spasm or physical change. These products were used medically as a dilator, but were also recommended by quacks for treating the usual array of medical ailments.[40] R.H. Bragdon made the similar Sphincter Muscle Expander. Benko's Adjustable Rectal Dilator could be adjusted in width by a screw mechanism. The Pneumatic Dilator was a rubber balloon that could be inflated after insertion by means of a hand-operated squeeze bulb.[41]

A further adaptation of these devices was the Recto Rotor Lubricating Dilator, a hard-rubber dilator produced by Lamothe Surgical Corporation. The dilator was inserted into the rectum to "massage the muscles of the rectal region."[42] Then, by rotating the knurled base, ointment was squeezed out of the tip. One of their advertisements stated, "The RECTO ROTOR is the only device that reaches the Vital Spot effectively."[43] The makers claimed "it would cure a man's lack of virility and give him high spirits and power." The Post Office shut the company down in 1932.

When electricity became a reality for medical treatment, dilators, such as these, were coupled with electric power to create heated probes that were inserted into the rectum and used to warm the prostate internally. Supposedly these products produced curative results due to heat applied directly to the source of the trouble. Similar treatments had been performed by legitimate physicians in the 1880s, but this was not done at home. These newer electrically-powered combination dilators and prostate warmers for home use offered much the same promise as the electric belt, namely improved sexual vigor and performance.

Two electrical products for gland warming were widely marketed between 1920 and 1940. In 1918 John G. Homan of Steubenville, Ohio, received a patent for a dilator manufactured by the Electrothermal Company, which combined pseudo-science about glands with electric technology to make the Thermalaid.[44] The Thermalaid was a hard-rubber rectal dilator and prostate gland warmer that was inserted into the rectum to apply heat to the prostate. The patent claimed, the device was intended to "excite the nerves and stimulate the capillary blood vessels." In a sweeping statement, the inventor claimed, "The reflex nerve action also has the effect of stimulating, through the so-called abdominal brain, those centers which have the tendency to bring about normal healthy conditions, thus relieving an aggravating cause of several diseases."[45]

The device provided heat to supposedly stimulate blood vessels and improve the "local nerve condition." The device plugged into the wall socket with an extension cord and used a 100-watt light bulb in the circuit to regulate the current and control the heat. The Thermalaid was available for use with available household electric current for $20, but if no electric service was available in the home, a separate battery-powered model was available for $25. The device was claimed to cure prostatic disease, and was also recommended as a cure for hemorrhoids.

The Electrothermal Company also made the Electro-thermal Vitalizer for use by women, to be inserted in the vagina. Sales were made primarily by advertising in newspapers and magazines. The FTC issued a cease-and-desist order for the devices in 1936.[46]

The Thermalaid was made to appear to be an outgrowth of the latest gland research, and advertising claimed that every man needed one if he had any kind of sexual dysfunction. As part of the product marketing, in 1923 the company published and distributed a book titled *Glands of Power and Success*, subtly appealing to every man's desire for success. Healthy glands were supposed to promote brain power, leanness, and youth. Unhealthy glands produced sexual dysfunction. An energized gland (produced by the Thermalaid, of course) was supposed to fill the user with health, vigor, and vitality.[47]

Another popular prostate warmer was the GHR Electric Thermitis Dilator, manufactured by GHR Electric Dilator Company of Grand Rapids, Michigan. Similar to the Thermalaid, it was advertised for use by both men and women.

The American Medical Association investigated all these devices and stated that prostate warmers were "more or less mechanical masturbation" devices. The use and popularity of these devices declined in the 1940s with a rising tide of homophobia in the country. As a result, any kind of anal penetration, even for medical purposes, raised fears of latent homosexuality.[48]

THIRTEEN

The Power
of Radioactivity

A nother scientific discovery that was ripe for medical fraud was
invisible radiation, when the discovery of radium and X-rays
in the 1890s brought the promise of unseen and powerful sources of
energy to treat disease. Scientists were fascinated by the energy potential of radium and they envisioned using this whole new source of
energy on the human body. Small amounts of radium seemed capable
of releasing large amounts of energy, and many believed that radium
could even power the body. Between 1900 and 1940 scientists, quacks,
and consumers struggled to turn radium into a fountain of youth and
described it, as they had electricity before it, as the ultimate energy cure.
Unfortunately, even scientists of the time did not understand the dangers of radiation and many ultimately died from the horrors of radium
poisoning.

At one time it had not seemed far-fetched that electricity could
drive disease out of the body, and now it was considered possible that
radium could provide a fountain of energy. Enthusiasts claimed that
radium could permanently energize the body through cellular renewal.
Some in the medical profession thought that radium worked by direct
application to the diseased parts. Others thought it stimulated the endocrine system, in particular the adrenal and thyroid glands.

Radium was not considered to be a drug, but a natural element,
thus it was not regulated as drugs were. The public had no reason to dis-
believe improbable sales pitches, and eager users were always willing to
provide testimonials about the efficacy of any new product. Boosted by
wild conjecture in articles and fiction in the popular press, the general

public easily believed that radium could invigorate the body and permanently boost physical and mental powers.

The Nature of Radiation

French physicist Henri Becquerel proposed the concept of radioactivity in 1896, when he observed that uranium fogged photographic plates and noted that mysterious unknown rays emanating from the substance could pass through skin and bone. Further work by Marie and Pierre Curie in Paris resulted in 1902 in the discovery and isolation of the element radium, a naturally-occurring substance in uranium ore.[1]

Scientists were fascinated by the potential of radioactive material because even small amounts of radium appeared to be capable of

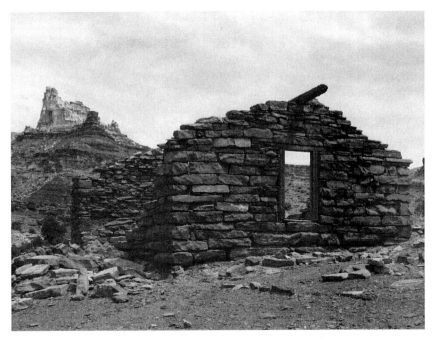

In the late 1800s researcher Marie Curie reportedly used uranium ore mined from Temple Mountain (in the background) in Utah for her studies of the treatment of cancer. Accounts from the period say that all the ore mined here was for her and was shipped to France. Local lore says that she stayed in this old miner's stone cabin when she visited Utah to inspect the source of her high-quality ore (author's collection).

releasing very large amounts of energy. Radium had a long half-life, and samples did not appear to decline in mass over a period of many years or in the amount of radiation emitted.[2] Fueled by wild speculation, the idea grew that radium could permanently create or boost physical and mental powers. It was a small jump in speculation to people believing that radium could invigorate the body.

Radioactive Hot Springs

Throughout the nineteenth century, bathing in hot springs was used as a treatment for intractable diseases such as tuberculosis and syphilis, and to treat temporary ailments such as dyspepsia and neurasthenia. Seeing a building enthusiasm for radium water, spas investigated the chemical contents of their springs. Some of the thermal springs in Europe that were tested were found to contain varying quantities of radioactive properties. Between 1910 and 1915 numerous American spas also "discovered" radium in their waters. Spas had previously touted the mineral content of their waters to legitimize medical claims, but after the discovery of radioactivity, the radioactive content of mineral water was promoted for health use. Wild claims emerged that radium helped to carry energy deeper into the body than electrotherapy. After a radium soak, cell activity was supposedly stimulated, secretory and excretory organs were aroused, and waste left the body rapidly. At the turn of the century electrical baths and electrical belts were felt to be the most effective way to put energy in the body, but now radium was promoted as regenerating the body at the cellular level.[3]

In the early 1920s patients were urged to use the *Radium Inhalatorium* at Bath, in England, to inhale radon gas from the spring water, in order to absorb as much radiation as possible.[4] Even the prestigious Battle Creek Sanitarium in Battle Creek, Michigan, had a special room where patients could inhale radium. Bathing in radioactive mud was also popular.

Dr. Basil Creighton, an early physician at the popular health spa in Manitou Springs, Colorado, placed high value on the medicinal use of radioactive water, saying, "Radio-active emanations have energizing and vivifying qualities which are stimulating to all cell activity. They endow fluid particles with active motility, thus promoting rapid absorption." He felt that individuals drinking radioactive mineral spring water would benefit in cases of "functional disorders of the stomach, gastric ulcers, systemic diseases as diabetes, Bright's engorgements of the liver, the anaemias, and conditions termed the uric acid diathesis." And "it was effective in catarrhal conditions of the nose and throat." He felt that bathing in this water was effective in cases of "obesity, gout, the neuroses, neurasthenia, gastritis, icterus, the various forms of rheumatism, sub-acute arthritis, incipient Bright's disease and incipient arterio-sclerosis."[5]

Mineral water advocates had always claimed that mineral water contained healing minerals that were not found in home tap water. In 1910 hydrotherapist Guy Hinsdale pointed out that waters containing a comparatively small amount of minerals had been claimed to have a therapeutic value which ordinary chemical analysis had failed to explain, and felt it was possible that the recent discovery of the radioactive properties of some of these waters might explain these healing qualities.[6]

Radium Water Dispensers

Scientists considered radium to have incredible amounts of energy locked up in its chemical atoms, so an illogical jump in reasoning by medical quacks was that this energy could be transferred to humans by ingesting radium. As a result, a popular craze developed in the 1920s for radium drinking water, thinking that the practice was healthy and curative. The ingestion of radium water, like treatments with electricity, was theorized to carry energy deep into the core of the body. Drinking radium water supposedly exposed the organs and glands to this amazing new source of energy that would add years to the lifespan. The typical recommended dosage was five or six glasses of water a day for sixty to ninety days in order to gain the full benefit of the energy and eliminate disease.[7] At the health spa at Rotorua in New Zealand, water containing radium was recommended for the treatment of gout, diabetes, and for the "tightening of loose teeth."

The easiest way to ingest radioactive water was with a radium water dispenser, which was a water jar with radium embedded in the interior surface. Many models of radium water dispenser were available. They included the Radium Vitalizer, the VigoRadium, the Radium Spa, the Radiumator, the Radium Ore Revigator, the Lifetime Radium Water Jar, the Radium Emanator, the Zimmer Emanator, Thomas's Radium Jars, the Radioak Generator, the Health Fountain from Radium-Health Corporation, and the Radium Vitalizer Generator. These devices supposedly created a perpetual radium health spring right in the user's home. Many of these were sold door-to-door, costing from about $8 to $15.

One of the popular devices to add radon to water was the Revigator radium water dispenser made by Radium Ore Revigator Company of San Francisco. The jar was invented by R.W. Thomas and first patented in 1912. It was simply a six-quart pottery jar lined with radioactive carnotite, a primary ore of uranium that emitted radon gas. As the uranium decomposed, it produced radon that was absorbed into the water.[8] The instructions were to fill the jar with water and drink six or seven glasses every day. Company advertising listed results from 10,011 cases treated, with 4,194 reporting that they were "cured," and 4,426 reporting that they had "benefited" from its use. As usual, the list of ailments that the water was claimed to treat covered almost everything. The unfortunate unmentioned side effect was that it also exposed drinkers to up to five times the amount of radium recommended for normal drinking water.

A typical testimonial for radium water came from J.D. Bright of Silver City, New Mexico, who complained, "My stomach and bowels seemed deranged and I was constipated, had no appetite and felt bad all the time." After drinking radium water he delightedly said, "I have improved from the first day that I began drinking the water and gained six pounds in weight. Appetite is fine and constipation is cured. My digestion is now perfect and I am sleeping sound."[9] Elderly enthusiast Franklin Ford, who had previously complained of rheumatism and feeling bad, claimed that after drinking radium water he could jump up and click his heels together.

Health, Vigor and Vitality

At the beginning of the twentieth century radium was regarded as a magic substance because its unseen powerful rays promised energy, plus it glowed in the dark. Legitimate scientists and quacks alike immediately pondered the question, what else could it do?

Scientists correctly realized that radium had unusual amounts of energy locked up in its chemical atoms; however, an illogical jump in reasoning was that this energy could be transferred to humans. As a result, radioactive ore was quickly added to many health products. Throughout the 1920s radium appeared in a variety of products, such as bath salts, beauty creams, mouthwash, ointments, face powder, and eyewashes. Radium toothpaste, radium hair tonic, and even radium-containing chocolate bars appeared on the market. In Grant County, New Mexico, Ra-Tor Mining and Manufacturing Company sold salves, toothpaste, and beauty products that were loaded with radium. The enthusiasm for radium was so great that a baker in Bath, in England, even baked "radium bread" for sale.[10]

Home Products Company of Denver, Colorado, formed in 1924, produced Vita Radium suppositories for men, ostensibly for treating prostate problems and issues of frequent urination, but also to rejuvenate sexual potency. The results promised were "restored glandular activity, sex-impulse and power; build-up of pep, personal magnetism and action; and raised resistance to colds." Similar "special suppositories" were available for vaginal insertion "for sexual apathy in women" to cure sexual afflictions and supposedly reinvigorate sexual desire.[11]

Typical of Home Products advertising was, "No matter whether you are old or young in years, if you are weak, you want STRENGTH! If you are feeling 'down and out,' you want of course to become PEPPY and ACTIVE again! If you are physically unfit for the duties and pleasures of a REAL MAN, you must long for a return of your normal, natural powers that fill life with joy, charm and happiness!" The advertisement continued on in a similar not-very-subtle theme.[12]

Home Products Company, operated by Dr. Davis and Marko Gacina, also made the Soothol Radium Boogie to treat premature ejaculation that they claimed may have been caused by "excessive indulgence, venereal infection and bad habits." The boogie was an eighth of an inch in diameter and six inches long, designed to be inserted into the male urethra. The recommended course of treatment was thirty days.

Home Products also made the Testone Radium Energizer and Suspensory, a radioactive belt that was worn like a diaper to direct radiation

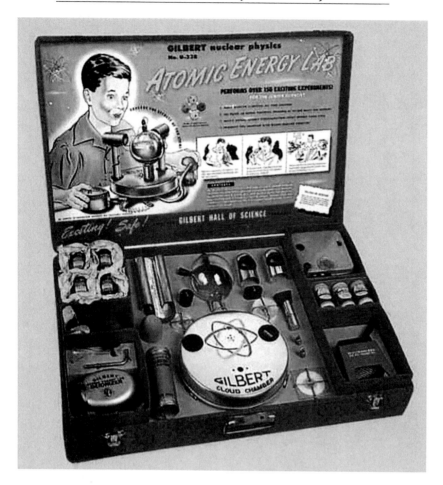

The Gilbert Atomic Energy Lab was a children's toy available from 1950 to 1951, when the Atomic Age was in its infancy. The actual risk of radiation to budding young scientists was probably minimal, but the set did include four small jars of radioactive material (on the upper left), including samples of uranium and radium. At one time called "the world's most dangerous toy," this chemistry set was later banned (Webms, Wikimedia Commons).

directly at the testicles. The company promised "new energy for weak sagging men." Again, not very subtle. In 1931 the company's products were finally judged to be fraudulent and barred from shipping through the mails.

Armbrecht, Nelson & Company of London offered special radium applicators, in the form of a slender rod with a radioactive tip, for insertion into the rectum or vagina to treat unspecified "problems."

The Radiendoctrinator

Radium was also incorporated in wearable devices, such as the Radiendoctrinator, invented by "Doctor" William J.A. Bailey. Bailey dropped out of college due to insufficient finances, but somewhere along the way supposedly picked up the title of "doctor" from the University of Vienna.

Bailey believed that aging was caused by a decline in function of the glands and that radiation would stimulate and revitalize them.[13] To do this, he developed the Radiendoctrinator, a gold-plated belt containing radium that produced gamma rays to "ionize the endocrine glands," thus increasing hormone production.[14]

The Radiendoctrinator was worn on different parts of the body, depending on what needed rejuvenation, and supposedly reinvigorated the thyroid, adrenals, the pituitary, the ovaries, or the prostate. If it was worn around the neck, it stimulated the thyroid. If worn around the waist, it worked on the adrenal glands. And if it was worn around the genitals as a suspensory pouch, it would hopefully rejuvenate the prostate. The belt was supposed to be worn for ten to thirty minutes, three or four times a day, though preferred treatment of the sex glands was overnight.

The Radiendoctrinator was manufactured in the late 1920s by American Endocrine Laboratories in New York City, which consisted of Bailey and Ward Leathers, with their associates Dr. Herman H. Rubin and Dr. C. Everett Field. Bailey had a previous conviction for fraud involving car sales.

In a 1924 address to the Medicinal Products of the American Chemical Society, Bailey claimed, "The wrinkled face, the drawn skin, the dull eye, the listless gait, the faulty memory, the aching body, the destructive effects of sterility, all spell imperfect endocrine performance." According to him the solution was to irradiate the glands. The specific way he did this was with two pads, two inches long by three inches wide, that attached to the body by a belt made of white satin and silk elastic. The pads were supposedly filled with radium, with a little mesotharium [sic] and actinium thrown in for good measure.[15]

The Radiendoctrinator sold originally for $1,000, but the effects of the Depression forced the price to drop in the 1930s to as low as $150.

The company shut itself down in the early 1930s rather than face fraud charges by the Post Office.

Bailey promoted three other radioactive products, the Bio-Ray which claimed to emit gamma rays for healing, and the Adrenoray, a belt containing five radioactive disks that was recommended for curing impotence, neurasthenia, and general debility, as well as the usual list of ailments. The third was a water irradiator called the Thoronator, a small vial that held two ounces of water in which there was a small cylinder that was said to give off thoron radiation that infused the water with radon gas.[16] In this manner tap water was supposedly transformed into radioactive water that was hundreds of times stronger than that produced by the old-fashioned radium jars. These products all disappeared in the 1930s, when concern for the safety of radioactive products became known.[17]

The Dangers of Radiation

Between 1900 and 1940 scientists, quacks, and consumers tried to turn radium into a fountain of youth. Few of the businessmen who jumped at the potential of radioactivity had any training in medicine and even fewer had any more than a casual layman's understanding of basic physics. Thus they were limited in their sales pitches by only their imaginations.

Even legitimate scientists investigating radioactivity did not understand the dangers of radiation. Several, such as pioneering scientist Marie Curie, eventually died from radium poisoning. She continued her work even though her health slowly declined, and she became weaker and weaker. Years of exposure to radiation weakened her body's red blood cells and she was eventually diagnosed as having a type of anemia. She refused, however, to believe that radium had anything to do with her illness. Another researcher, Henry Green, in spite of tiredness and sloughing skin, believed that his work with radium was necessary to keep up his energy level.[18]

On the layman's side, dangerous radioactive patent medicines were popular from about 1910 to the late 1930s. Promoters claimed that they transferred energy into the body from external radioactive sources and thus created new energy within the body. The dangers of this form of radium came to the forefront of consumer consciousness with the case of Eben M. Byers, who consumed daily large doses of a product called Radithor. Though Radithor falls more into the category of patent medicine, it will be discussed briefly here as it relates to Bailey and the dangers of radiation.

In 1925 William Bailey founded Bailey Radium Laboratories in East Orange, New Jersey, and between 1925 and 1930 sold Radithor, a liquid radium solution in a bottle. The sales pitch was that this radium elixir deposited radium into the body so that it could treat every cell. For those concerned with sexual potency, it would supposedly rejuvenate the body to a peak of capacity with every "gland" functioning at top efficiency. Bailey claimed that Radithor was excellent for sexual rejuvenation and that it would even cure the mentally ill. He hinted at an internal fountain of youth. Radithor was also supposed to benefit dyspepsia, high blood pressure, and impotence. But Radithor also contained two isotopes of radium, both of which emitted dangerously high levels of radiation.

Radithor was a profitable product as it cost Bailey an estimated twenty-five cents and each bottle sold for a dollar. Between 1925 and 1930 Bailey Radium Laboratories sold 400,000 bottles of Radithor. Eventually radiation toxicity led to an investigation.

In 1927, industrialist, steel tycoon, and millionaire Eben Byers suffered from lingering pain in his arm due to a serious injury received during a train accident. His physician prescribed Radithor. Bailey claimed that this new radium drink he was taking had decreased the pain in his arm and increased his vitality. He further envisioned that it could create a perpetual internal fountain of youth. Byers was very enthusiastic about the product and started drinking three bottles a day. Between 1927 and 1930 he was estimated to have drunk 1,400 bottles of Radithor.

Predictably, Byers became extremely ill. His initial aches and pains were misdiagnosed and it wasn't until too late that his doctors realized that he was dying from radiation poisoning. His health gradually deteriorated as he continued to take large doses of Radithor, even as he suffered from the horrible effects of radiation poisoning. Four years later the large amounts of radium in his system resulted in a gruesome death.[19] The Federal Trade Commission started investigating Bailey's Company in 1928, but it was not until 1931 that they were able to complete their investigation and issued a cease-and-desist order.

As the dangers of radioactivity became evident, all these radioactive products were eventually withdrawn from the market and radium was banned from medicines and personal products.

X-rays from Head to Toe

William Konrad Roentgen, a German physicist, discovered X-rays in late 1895. He named the mysterious radiation the X-ray, because of its unknown character. The invisible ray allowed physicians to see inside the body to detect foreign objects, and inspect damaged organs and broken bones. For the first time it was possible to look inside the human body without surgery or other invasive methods, and X-rays were soon being used to diagnose a wide range of conditions. Similar to radium, however, the dangerous nature of X-rays and using them on the body was not understood.[20]

In the late 1940s and early 1950s, X-ray machines were commonly used in shoe stores for fitting shoes. This was a fluoroscope that was used to help people try on shoes by visualizing if the shoes fit properly. The first machine was developed by Boston physician Jacob Lowe, who received a patent on his invention, the Foot-O-Scope, in 1927.[21]

The machine consisted of a wooden cabinet, about the size of a modern dishwasher, with an X-ray generator at the bottom and a fluoroscope screen above it. The customer put his or her feet into a slot at the base of the unit. The machine was turned on and X-rays penetrated the feet and shoes, producing an image of the feet inside the shoes. There were three viewing ports on top of the cabinet. One for the customer to view their feet as a ghostly green translucent image on the screen, one for the salesman to comment on the fit, and one for a mother or spouse to be part of the fitting. All three could see how the feet fit and moved inside the shoe.

Eventually an estimated 10,000 devices were in use in shoe and department stores at a cost of $2,000 each. The dominant company that manufactured the machines was the Adrian X-ray Company of Milwaukee.

By the 1950s these devices were recognized to be a radiation hazard. Part of this was due to high levels of radiation that leaked from the machine and some was due to faulty adjustment of the X-ray mechanism. In 1953 the Foot-O-Scope and Pedoscope were banned by the Federal Government.[22] By 1970 all foot X-ray machines were essentially banned.

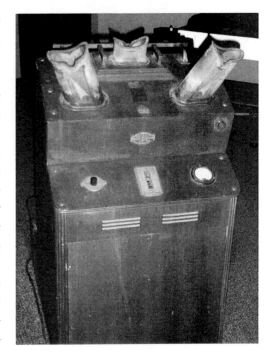

Another dangerous source of radiation was this shoe X-ray device, commonly used for fitting shoes on children. The machine contained three viewing ports, one for the wearer to look through at his or her feet, one for mother to check the fit, and one for the shoe salesman to reinforce the sale. Unfortunately the unintended result was that at the same time all three received large doses of radiation. This shoe fluoroscope was manufactured around 1938 by Adrian Shoe Fitter, Inc. (National Museum of Health and Medicine).

Another dangerous use for X-rays from the late 1920s to the 1940s was for the removal of unwanted hair. One such device was the Tricho hair removal system. Similar manufacturers were the Dermic Institute, the EpiaX-ray, Hair-X Laboratories, and the Hamomar Method and Marton Method. The Tricho machine was developed by Dr. Albert C. Geyser, professor of physiological therapy and chief of clinic at Fordham University, and chief of the electro and roentgenray clinic at Cornell College. His theory was that by totally treating the skin at one time all the hair follicles would be destroyed at the same time, thus removing unwanted hair. He was a medical doctor and a scientist with impressive credentials, but he did not seem to understand the dangers of radiation. Typical users were young women from their late teens and early twenties who believed the company advertising claims that young men found excess body hair to be a deterrent to marriage.

Warnings about the dangers of exposure to X-rays started to appear in medical journals in the late 1920s. The unfortunate side effects of X-ray treatment for hair removal were hardened and wrinkled skin, receding gums, sores on the face and legs, and cancer. In 1929, the American Medical Association started to publish reports of injuries caused by the Tricho device. Nevertheless, the Tricho stayed on the market and thousands of patients were exposed to dangerous X-rays simply in the name of beauty.

Postscript

The second half of the nineteenth century was a time of discoveries and changes that resulted in major medical innovations to cure diseases and conditions that were previously deadly. Even though the first half of the twentieth century was a time of rapid development of modern medicine and surgery, about 90 percent of the modern medical miracles that we take for granted today date from the end of World War II in 1945. It was not until the early 1940s, for example, that researchers realized the potential of penicillin for killing bacteria, and only during the last few years of World War II was enough penicillin produced to treat men wounded in battle.

The list of medical achievements since 1945 is impressive. Heart, liver, and lung transplants are possible. Powerful new drugs combat cancer and AIDS. The development of machines for kidney dialysis has extended the life of people with failing kidneys. Oral contraceptives, first perfected in the 1950s, offer women precise control of family planning.

Beyond the use of X-rays, several other radical new methods have been developed for imaging the inside of the human body. Ultrasonic imaging uses high frequency sound waves to see internal organs. Thermography detects and analyzes minute temperature differences in tissues to detect cancer tumors and arthritic joints. Computer axial tomography (CAT) combines X-rays with computer analysis to create a three-dimensional view of sections of the internal organs. Magnetic resonance imaging (MRI) uses a powerful magnetic field to excite hydrogen atoms in the body to create a three-dimensional image of soft tissues. Fiber optic endoscopes inserted into body openings allow detailed direct viewing of the inside of the urinary and gastrointestinal tracts.

Legitimate Use of Electricity

Legitimate electronic devices, such as the electrocardiogram (EKG) for measuring heart waves and the electroencephalogram (EEG) for measuring brain waves are useful and legitimate medical devices. In the early 1990s the use of electricity was investigated for the prevention of osteoporosis and as a possible way to help heal bone. One hospital in Pennsylvania has tested the use of a Tesla coil to produce an electric field that might help to stimulate endorphins.

Electric shocks and levels of electrical current that burned faded away as a method of treatment in the 1920s. Electricity, however, is still useful for certain treatments. The use of electrotherapy to relieve pain is the basis of today's Transcutaneous Electrical Nerve Stimulation (TENS) devices, which send a small electric current through the skin. These devices can be very effective in cases of intractable pain, such as inoperable back pain.

Control at Last

When the U.S. Food and Drug Administration began to regulate medical devices in 1938, the agency had to prove that a product was unsafe or fraudulent before taking action against the manufacturer. There was no way to prevent unsafe or ineffective devices from coming onto the market, and any regulatory or legal action had to take place after the fact.

In 1976 Congress passed the Medical Devices Amendments to the Food, Drug, and Cosmetic Act to require that new medical devices were safe and effective before going on the market. For the first time, the Medical Device Amendments placed the burden of proof on the manufacturer. Previously the law was limited to action against hazardous or falsely-represented devices after they went on sale.

In 1990 the law was further amended with the Safe Medical Devices Act (SMDA), which gave the FDA increased powers to prosecute manufacturers of dubious medical devices, and required medical facilities and product distributors to report to the FDA the number of adverse effects, including deaths, serious illnesses, and serious injuries, related to medical devices. In spite of these efforts, people still spend large amounts of money each year on untested and quack medical cures that will not help them.

In spite of increased legislation, fraudulent medical devices still find their way into the marketplace. In the mid–1990s a device named The Stimulator, made by Universal Management Service of Akron, Ohio, claimed that it could cure pain from menstrual problems and arthritis. It was basically a BBQ gas-grill igniter that applied a spark to the skin when the user pushed a plunger that struck a crystal to generate electricity. The FDA filed an injunction. Others, however, were quick to jump on the bandwagon with the Crystaldyne Pain Reliever sold from Scottsdale, the Piezo D-X Quartz Crystal from Bright Marketing in Ohio, and the Acupoint Pulse Stimulator from Magna Plus of Ohio.

Another example of consumer beware was the series of Hieronymus machines, invented by electrical engineer Thomas Galen Hieronymus, who claimed to use the same radionic principles developed by Albert Abrams eighty years before. The best-known Hieronymus Machine is the Eloptic Medical Analyzer, which supposedly analyzes and transmits "eloptic energy" (a combination of electrical and optical energy) to diagnose and treat medical conditions. Eloptic radiation has never been detected by scientific instruments and there is no other evidence of its existence, so the scientific community has been skeptical at best.

Others included the BT-7 "Brain Tuner," which was an electronic stimulator that was claimed to produce over five hundred frequencies that rapidly balanced and restored the natural energies of the body and mind. Their advertising offered an improved ability to focus, enhanced creativity, reduced nervous energy, better sexual performance, and increased mental and physical energy. It was sold on the Internet at a cost of $175. Microwater ionizers operate to produce water that is supposedly antioxidant-rich with concentrated alkaline minerals that facilitate the rapid absorption of food nutrients. Because microwater has a higher concentration of alkaline minerals, it is allegedly far more effective at detoxifying the body of harmful acid waste.

A casual search on the internet will show that quite a few of the devices mentioned in this book as historical devices have reappeared in modern form. As recently as 1970s, for example, a modernized metal version of the Resuscitator was being sold in Germany for producing "health through skin irritation treatment." The use of electric currents driven through the skin is used in modern TENS devices. Dry cupping is still legitimately used today to promote blood flow in the capillaries of the skin, but the modern version uses a vacuum pump to achieve the same result. Vibrating exercise devices are sold on late-night television for weight reduction and toning the muscles. A cap similar to the Thermocap from the 1920s, lined with tiny light sources to stimulate the growth of hair, is being sold on television. A modern version of Tyrrell's J.B.L. Cascade device is available via mail order, along with Young's Dilators. And at least two modern versions of the electrically-powered prostate warmer are available for purchase via the Internet.

Today most fraudulent devices are off the market. An enhanced FDA pre-market approval process and post-market controls, along with additional governmental regulatory authority over devices, has help to keep dangerous or harmful devices away from the public. However, unconventional devices appear from time to time, often sold on television or the Internet, just as charlatans previously used advertisements in cheap periodicals and sold through mail order. Though government regulations of medical devices mostly protect us from ourselves, it is still a case of "Consumer Beware."

Glossary:
Medical Terminology

The following are not all-encompassing definitions, but are intended as an explanation of some of the medical terms that appear in the text, some of which are used in the context of nineteenth-century medicine and may have slightly different meanings today.

Arthritis: inflammation of a body joint due to various conditions. Usually accompanied by pain.

Autointoxication: a theory that a lack of frequent bowel movements resulted in toxic products in the large intestine being reabsorbed into the body and causing illness. This unfounded belief became a national worry and obsession from about 1880 until the 1930s.

Bacteria: one-celled living micro-organisms that can produce disease. Bacteria can typically be killed in the body by antibiotics or on surfaces by chemical disinfectants.

Bilious: an archaic term for symptoms of a disordered liver used as a catch-all name, particularly by manufacturers of patent medicines, for any vague feelings of physical discomfort, such as tiredness, headache, constipation, or loss of appetite.

Bleeding: one of the primary treatments used in Heroic Medicine, in which a physician deliberately cut into a vein and allowed blood to drain out of the body, in the theory that this would relieve the "morbid excitement" and congestion that was causing fever and disease.

Bougie: a slender metal or rubber tubular instrument for exploring and dilating body canals, such as the urethra.

Calomel: mercurous chloride (chloride of mercury, also called horn mercury or sweet mercury) used for purging the bowels and treating syphilis. Mercury was poisonous and its continued use induced various serious neurological problems, nevertheless calomel was one of the most frequently prescribed drugs in nineteenth-century therapeutics.

Catarrh: an older generic medical term that was used to describe any inflammation of the mucus membranes of the breathing organs, such as in the throat and lungs.

Cathartic: a medicine that produces a series of violent bowel evacuations, often accompanied by pain and cramping. One of the most frequently prescribed drugs in nineteenth-century therapeutics was calomel (mercurous chloride), commonly used in Heroic Medicine for purging the bowels.

Chlorosis: in the nineteenth century the term was often used interchangeably with hysteria. The more modern meaning refers to a form of iron-deficiency anemia, particularly in young women, also called "greensickness," because the skin took on a greenish pallor. This form of chlorosis is no longer seen because of modern improved nutrition and adequate iron in the diet.

Cholera: a severe gastrointestinal infection transmitted by a bacterium and spread through contaminated water and food supplies. Major cholera epidemics raged through the United States in 1832, 1849, and 1866.

Clyster: an antiquated medical term that generally referred to an enema, though the term clyster was also used generically to include the injection of healing substances into all of the body cavities, such as the ear, nose, bladder, and uterus. Older medical texts sometimes spell this as "glyster."

Colonic Irrigation: flushing the intestinal tract with large volumes of water in order to thoroughly cleanse the internal system. Under various names this treatment was adopted by almost all the Victorian spas as an important form of treatment for dyspepsia and autointoxication.

Colonic Lavage: another name for *Colonic Irrigation*.

Consumption: a Victorian term for tuberculosis, caused by the bacillus *Mycobacterium tuberculosis*, spread by an infected person's cough. Another older name was the "white plague" for the white spongy material that formed in the lungs.

Costiveness: an antiquated medical term for constipation.

Douche: in Victorian medicine this term was used to describe high-pressured jets of hot or cold water that were applied to the outside of the body by various means. The more modern meaning describes an irrigation of the vagina. The Victorian medical term for the latter was *Vaginal Injection*.

Dropsy: An older term for the accumulation of fluid in the body due to congestive heart failure.

Dyspepsia: indigestion (which is a synonym) arising from various causes, such as disease, excessive use of alcohol, or dietary indiscretion. Not a disease in itself, but a symptom of other disorders.

Electrotherapy: the application of electrical current to treat various medical conditions.

Emetic: a substance that produces vomiting.

Enema: the apparatus or procedure for injecting water or various drugs into the bowel through the anus for the purposes of cleansing or medicating.

Fleam: essentially the same as a *Lancet*.

Greensickness: see *Chlorosis*.

Hard Rubber: a product of the vulcanization of natural rubber by heating it with sulfur. If the process was carried to an extreme, the resulting hard material was called "hard rubber," also known as vulcanite, used for manufacturing various medical devices.

Heroic Medicine: medical treatments based on humoral theory, consisting primarily of bleeding, purging, blistering, vomiting, and sweating to supposedly remove toxic material and rebalance the humors.

Homeopathic Medicine: a system of medicine that treated illness through highly diluted concentrations of drugs that induced the symptoms of the disease.

Humoral Theory: ancient Greek medical theory that the body contained four fluids called humors, consisting of blood (*sanguis*), phlegm (*pituita*), yellow bile (*chole*), and black bile (*melanchole*). These humors corresponded to the four material elements of air, water, fire, and earth; and four conditions of hot, wet, cold, and dry. Good health was considered to depend on the balance of the four humors, and illness supposedly meant that the humors were out of balance.

Hydriatics: the treatment of disease with large amounts of water, both external and internal; a synonym for *Hydrotherapy*.

Hydropathy: even though technically incorrect, this term, which literally means "water disease," was commonly used to describe the treatment of disease with large amounts of water, both externally and internally, typically as cold baths and high pressure showers. This type of therapy should more correctly be called *Hydrotherapy*, which means "water treatment."

Hydrotherapy: the treatment of various ailments via the use of water applied to the body externally and internally.

Hygeiotherapy: a newer name for *Hydropathy* that was developed in the 1850s with the idea that improved hygiene could treat, cure, and maintain health.

Hysteria: an imprecise clinical diagnosis derived from the Greek name for the womb, used in Victorian medicine to describe a series of nebulous symptoms in women that could be related to almost every type of physical disease. Symptoms would be termed "hysterical neurosis" by psychotherapists. After 1895, when Drs. Josef Breuer and Sigmund Freud published *Studies in Hysteria*, the specific disease passed into the realm of psychoanalysis and eventually faded from the medical scene as a specific ailment.

Injection: prior to the introduction of hypodermic injections in 1853 to deliver medicine directly under the skin, the term "injection" was used to describe an enema. "Throwing up an injection" was an antiquated term for administering an enema. Another Victorian term used in the water-cure establishments was *Lavement*.

Intestinal Lavage: a less-threatening alternative term adopted to describe the popular spa treatment of *Colonic Irrigation*, first introduced at the spa at Plombières, France, as the *Plombières Douche*.

Lancet: A sharp pointed surgical knife with two edges, used for bleeding a patient. The leading British medical journal, *The Lancet*, is named after this instrument.

Lavage: another name for **Colonic Irrigation**.

Laxative: a drug used to induce a bowel movement.

Neuralgia: severe pain associated with a nerve.

Neurasthenia: a nebulous and ill-defined mental "disease" of men, with symptoms similar to hysteria in women. It exhibited symptoms of multiple diseases without any organic cause and was accompanied by fatigue, weakness, irritability, an inability to concentrate, and various aches and pains.

Phrenology: a pseudo-science concerned with the study of the shape of the head in the belief that its bumps could be used to predict the character and intellectual traits of an individual.

Placebo: an inactive substance or a treatment with no intrinsic therapeutic value, but which can produce a sense of relief and healing power in a patient through the powers of suggestion, reassurance, and imagination.

Psychosomatic Illness: a pathological condition due to mental or emotional factors with no discoverable basis in physical illness.

Purgative: a powerful laxative drug that produced a series of violent bowel evacuations.

Purging: one of the primary methods of treatment used in Heroic Medicine in which strong drugs were administered to a patient to make the bowels work vigorously under the theory that this would flush from the body any undesirable noxious material that was causing disease.

Rheumatism: a generic term applied to acute and chronic complaints characterized by stiffness and soreness in the muscles and pain in the joints, including arthritis.

Scarificator: an instrument used for bleeding that contained multiple spring-loaded blades that made multiple small incisions in the skin.

Solitary Vice: a polite Victorian name for masturbation; as opposed to the "social vices," which were adultery, fornication, and other forms of unlawful sexual intercourse.

Spa: a resort using mineral springs for treatment of various ailments. Spas also used heat, light, baths, various applications of water, massage, exercise, and diet as part of their treatment plans.

Spondylotherapy: a system of medicine that treated disease through spinal manipulation.

Subluxation: a partial dislocation between bones, such as in the spine, where some degree of contact is preserved.

Sudorific: A medicine intended to promote sweating; specifically, an agent that causes drops of perspiration to appear on the skin.

Tuberculosis: a widespread disease in the second half of the nineteenth century due to poor nutrition and crowded living conditions. The disease, more commonly known in Victorian times as "consumption" or "white plague," was contracted by direct contact, from inhaling bacteria-laden air, or by swallowing bacteria in food or drink.

Typhoid: also known as "malignant bilious fever" or "slow fever," was a severe infection caused by a bacterium that was not identified until 1880. Typhoid was transmitted through improperly prepared food or contact with contaminated water supplies.

Vapors: an obsolete vague term that applied to hysterical symptoms or imaginary illness in women.

Water-Cure: treatment of disease with large amounts of water, applied both externally and internally. The precursor of the spa and health sanitarium, the water-cure was popular from around 1820 to 1860.

Appendix:
The Electromagnetic Spectrum

Energy that travels via wave motion, known as radiant energy, extends over a wide range of frequencies. At the low end of the spectrum are sound waves that are audible to the human ear. At the upper end are cosmic rays that travel to (and through) us from outer space. In between is a variety of energy, including the visible spectrum that we can detect with our eyes and X-rays that are powerful enough to penetrate the human body. Various types of energy interact with and have been applied to the human body.

In ascending order of frequency, the radiant energy spectrum consists of:

Name	Uses/Effects
Audible frequencies (AF)	sound, human hearing, and speech communication
Radio waves (RF)	radio communication, television, microwave ovens, cell phones, GPS, radar
Infrared (IR)	penetrating body heating
Visible light	vision, lighting, seeing *the colors of the rainbow: red, orange, yellow, green, blue, violet*
Ultraviolet light (UV)	the cause of sunburn and skin cancer
X-rays	visualizing the internal structures of the body
Gamma rays (a by-product of natural radioactivity)	cancer therapy and diagnostic imaging
Cosmic rays	radiation from outer space

Chapter Notes

Chapter One

1. Oneill, *Unmentionable*, 261.
2. Janik, *Marketplace of the Marvelous*, 15.
3. Peña, *The Body Electric*, 96.
4. Steele, *Bleed, Blister and Purge*, 151.
5. Janik, *Marketplace of the Marvelous*, 245.
6. Kang and Pedersen, *Quackery*, 134.
7. Sutcliffe and Duin, *A History of Medicine*, 27.
8. Sutcliffe and Duin, *A History of Medicine*, 26.
9. Toledo-Pereyra, *A History of American Medicine*, 29.
10. Rutkow, *Seeking the Cure*, 32.
11. Armstrong and Armstrong, *The Great American Medicine Show*, 9.
12. Rutkow, *Seeking the Cure*, 17.
13. Rutkow, *Seeking the Cure*, 45.
14. Sutcliffe and Duin, *A History of Medicine*, 88.
15. Janik, *Marketplace of the Marvelous*, 188–189.
16. Toledo-Pereyra, *A History of American Medicine*, 100–101.
17. Whorton, *Nature Cures*, 168–169.

Chapter Two

1. Porter, *Quacks*, 11.
2. Sutcliffe and Duin, *A History of Medicine*, 42.
3. Porter, *The Greatest Benefit to Mankind*, 284.
4. Porter, *Quacks*, 90.
5. Quoted in Porter, *Quacks*, 98.
6. Thompson, *Counterknowledge*, 71.
7. Porter, *Quacks*, 15.
8. McCoy, *Quack*, 21.

9. McCoy, *Quack*, 20.
10. Washington, Pennsylvania *Observer-Reporter*, Mar 29, 1973.
11. *FDA Consumer*, Sep 1975, 33.
12. Cramp, *Nostrums and Quackery*, 258.
13. Dary, *Frontier Medicine*, 278, 289.
14. Kang and Pedersen, *Quackery*, v.
15. Steele, *Bleed, Blister and Purge*, 152.
16. Holbrook, *The Golden Age of Quackery*, 241.
17. Janik, *Marketplace of the Marvelous*, 200.
18. Steele, *Bleed, Blister and Purge*, 156.
19. Section 201(h) of the Food, Drug & Cosmetic Act; 21 U.S. Code § 321.
20. For readers seeking further specific information on federal regulations, medical devices are controlled by the Code of Federal Regulations, Title 21, which consists of nine volumes, each of which are revised at least once each calendar year. Most of the volumes concern the regulation of food, drugs, and cosmetics. Medical devices are described in Volume 8, parts 800 to 1299. Most devices fall into one of three categories. Class I (low risk) devices, which require only general controls; Class II (medium risk) devices, which require pre-market approval and have written mandatory performance standards; and Class III (high risk) devices, such as pacemakers, which require pre-market approval from the FDA.

Chapter Three

1. Thompson, *Counterknowledge*, 1.
2. Gardner, *Fads and Fallacies in the Name of Science*, 186.
3. Whorton, *Nature Cures*, 6.

4. K.B. Thomas, "General Practice Consultations: Is There a Point in Being Positive," *British Medical Journal*, 294, 1987, 1200–1202.

5. Gant, *Constipation and Intestinal Obstruction*, 206.

6. Janik, *Marketplace of the Marvelous*, 263.

7. Cynthia Crossen, *Tainted Truth: The Manipulation of Fact in America* (New York: Simon & Schuster, 1994), 176.

8. Walter A. Brown, "The Placebo Effect," *Scientific American*, Jan 1998, 90–95.

9. Thompson, *Counterknowledge*, 74.

10. Gant, *Constipation and Intestinal Obstruction*, 212.

11. Janik, *Marketplace of the Marvelous*, 264.

12. Gant, *Constipation and Intestinal Obstruction*, 228.

13. *FDA Consumer Magazine*, Jan-Feb 2000.

14. Gant, *Constipation and Intestinal Obstruction*, 213.

15. Coolidge, *Statistics*, 25.

16. Rumsey, *Statistics for Dummies*, 57.

17. Coolidge, *Statistics*, 10.

18. Rumsey, *Statistics for Dummies*, 275.

19. Coolidge, *Statistics*, 328.

20. Coolidge, *Statistics*, 135.

Chapter Four

1. Warren, *Old Medical and Dental Instruments*, 4.

2. Warren, *Old Medical and Dental Instruments*, 7.

3. Warren, *Old Medical and Dental Instruments*, 27.

4. Edna M. Bennett and John F. Bennett, *Turquoise Jewelry of the Indians of the Southwest* (Colorado Springs, CO: Turquoise Books, 1973), 12.

5. Porter, *Quacks*, 68–69.

6. Porter, *Quacks*, 101.

7. Belofsky, *Strange Medicine*, 142.

8. Steele, *Bleed, Blister and Purge*, 162–163.

9. Belofsky, *Strange Medicine*, 48.

10. Green, *Fit for America*, 4.

11. Kang and Pedersen, *Quackery*, 133.

12. The prestigious British medical journal *The Lancet* was named after the tool.

13. Warren, *Old Medical and Dental Instruments*, 16.

14. Georgiana J. Sanders, *Modern Methods in Nursing* (Philadelphia: W.B. Saunders, 1917), 143–144.

15. Warren, *Old Medical and Dental Instruments*, 16.

16. Sanders, *Modern Methods in Nursing*, 145–146.

17. Child, *The Family Nurse*, 76.

18. Morris, *The Mystery of the Exploding Teeth*, 107.

19. Russell, *Colonic Irrigation*, 6.

20. Morris, *The Mystery of the Exploding Teeth*, 110–111.

21. Kang and Pedersen, *Quackery*, 50–51.

22. E. Hutchinson, *Ladies' Indispensable Assistant* (New York: no publisher, 1851), 32.

23. Child, *The Family Nurse*, 76.

24. Morris, *The Mystery of the Exploding Teeth*, 113.

25. Holbrook, *The Golden Age of Quackery*, 35.

26. Gardner, *Fads and Fallacies in the Name of Science*, 204.

27. Holbrook, *The Golden Age of Quackery*, 35.

28. It is difficult to state the value of money in 1790 in today's terms and purchasing power. This amount is roughly equivalent in buying power to $600 today, but this figure cannot necessarily be considered to be an equivalent worth. In terms of value in 1790, however, this was the price of a cow or the wages of a skilled laborer for a month.

29. McCoy, *Quack*, 27.

30. Holbrook, *The Golden Age of Quackery*, 36.

31. McCoy, *Quack*, 28.

32. Holbrook, *The Golden Age of Quackery*, 35.

33. McCoy, *Quack*, 28.

34. Hart-Davis, *What the Victorians Did for Us*, 157.

35. The name "rubber" was initially applied to the soft, sticky sap that came from the rubber tree that grows in tropical countries. Charles Goodyear developed a process to cure India rubber by heating it with sulfur to create the soft latex rubber used for rubber gloves and other medical devices. If the process was carried further, the rubber became solid and the resulting hard material was called "hard rubber," known also as "vulcanite."

36. Hart-Davis, *What the Victorians Did for Us*, 141–142.

37. Whorton, *Nature Cures*, 259–261.

38. Whorton, *Nature Cures*, 270.

39. Whorton, *Nature Cures*, 261–262.

40. Warren, *Old Medical and Dental Instruments*, 20.

41. Belofsky, *Strange Medicine*, 156.

42. Ronald Melzack and Joel Katz, "Auriculotherapy fails to relieve chronic pain. A controlled crossover study," *Journal of the American Medical Association*, 251(8), 1984, 1041–1043.

43. Pierre Rabischong and Claudie Terral, "Scientific Basis of Auriculotherapy: State of the Art," *Medical Acupuncture*, 26 (2), Apr 1, 2014, 84–96.

44. As an interesting side note, words in our vocabulary such as "highbrow" and "lowbrow" originated with phrenology.

45. Janik, *Marketplace of the Marvelous*, 55.

46. McCoy, *Quack*, 135.

47. Janik, *Marketplace of the Marvelous*, 58.

48. Janik, *Marketplace of the Marvelous*, 61.

49. Fowler and Fowler, *The Illustrated Self-Instructor in Phrenology and Physiology*, frontispiece illustration.

50. Whorton, *Nature Cures*, 97.

51. Janik, *Marketplace of the Marvelous*, 68.

52. McCoy, *Quack*, 12.

53. McCoy, *Quack*, 142–143.

54. Janik, *Marketplace of the Marvelous*, 78.

Chapter Five

1. Thatcher advertisement in *The Poultry Keeper*, 1885, 207.

2. Advertisement from Prof. Chas. Bidwell Manufacturing Company, Chicago, 1922.

3. McCoy, *Quack*, 33.

4. Peña, *The Body Electric*, 4.

5. Walsh, *Cures*, 78–80.

6. Scientifically speaking, there is no such thing as the ether. In the seventeenth and eighteenth centuries, the ether (also spelled aether) was thought to be a substance that supposedly filled all of space above the earth to explain the propagation of electromagnetic and gravitational forces. This theory was proved to be scientifically incorrect, as the development of the theory of special relativity showed that the ether is not required for the transmission of this energy.

7. Whorton, *Nature Cures*, 104; Lara Owen, *Pain Free with Magnet Therapy* (New York: Three Rivers Press, 2000), 21.

8. However, remember the earlier comments about statistical significance in Chapter Three. It can be said that Mesmer based much of his work on an initial sample of one, rather than on a proper statistical experiment.

9. Armstrong and Armstrong, *The Great American Medicine Show*, 188.

10. Janik, *Marketplace of the Marvelous*, 153.

11. Franz Mesmer, *Maxims on Animal Magnetism* (Mt. Vernon, NY: Eden Press, 1958), 76.

12. Margolis, *The Intimate History of the Orgasm*, 258.

13. Whorton, *Nature Cures*, 107.

14. Armstrong and Armstrong, *The Great American Medicine Show*, 188.

15. Sutcliffe and Duin, *A History of Medicine*, 43.

16. Janik, *Marketplace of the Marvelous*, 156.

17. Whorton, *Nature Cures*, 109–112.

18. Joseph C. Furnas, *The Life and Times of the Late Demon Rum* (New York: Capricorn Books, 1973), 314.

19. Wroebel, *Pseudo-Science and Society in Nineteenth-Century America*, 5.

20. A few representative publications are: *Healing with Magnets* (Carroll & Graf, 1998) by Gary Null; *Magnet Therapy: The Pain Cure Alternative* (Prima Lifestyles, 1998) by Ron Lawrence, Paul J. Rosch, and Judith Plowden; and *Pain Free with Magnet Therapy* (Three Rivers Press, 2000) by Lara Owen.

21. McCoy, *Quack*, 40.

Chapter Six

1. Hart-Davis, *What the Victorians Did for Us*, 47.

2. Watkins, *A Manual of Electrotherapy*, 14.

3. Watkins, *A Manual of Electrotherapy*, 48.

4. Green, *Fit for America*, 72–73.

5. Watkins, *A Manual of Electrotherapy*, 14.

6. Watkins, *A Manual of Electrotherapy*, 240.

7. Rolls, *Diseased, Douched and Doctored*, 48.

8. J. J. Lowke, "Theory of electrical breakdown in air—the Role of Metastable Oxygen Molecules," *Journal of Physics D: Applied Physics*, 25 (2), 1992, 202–210.

9. Watkins, *A Manual of Electrotherapy*, 240.

10. Hart-Davis, *What the Victorians Did for Us*, 49.

11. Watkins, *A Manual of Electrotherapy*, 241.

12. Armstrong and Armstrong, *The Great American Medicine Show*, 186.

13. Rolls, *Diseased, Douched and Doctored*, 48.

14. Hart-Davis, *What the Victorians Did for Us*, 49.

15. Hart-Davis, *What the Victorians Did for Us*, 52.

16. In correct technical terms, current is produced by the movement of electrons in a conductor and electron flow from the negative terminal to the positive terminal of a battery. This sort of detail is beyond this brief discussion, and historical convention says that electrical current flows from the positive terminal to the negative terminal.

17. Alternating current is also described by the number of alternations that take place every second. Alternating current supplied to the wall socket or a light bulb in a house alternates, or reverses direction, sixty time per second, and thus is referred to as a frequency of 60 cycles-per-second or 60 Hertz, named after the German physicist Heinrich Hertz, who was the first to provide proof of electromagnetic waves.

18. Ari Davis was an inventor and craftsman, who patented the machine in 1854. Walter Kidder was a physician from Lowell, Massachusetts, who sold it.

19. Peña, *The Body Electric*, 96–97.

20. Saline solution, water with a little salt dissolved in it, is an excellent conductor of electricity.

21. Souter, *The Doctor's Bag*, 294.

22. For an extended discussion on professional use versus home use of medical batteries see: Anna Wexler, "The Medical Battery in The United States (1870–1920): Electrotherapy at Home and in the Clinic," *Journal of the History of Medicine and Allied Sciences*, 72 (2), Apr 2017, 166–192.

23. Maines, *The Technology of Orgasm*, 104.

24. Green, *Fit for America*, 168.

25. Watkins, *A Manual of Electrotherapy*, 141–142.

26. Watkins, *A Manual of Electrotherapy*, 168.

27. Peña, *The Body Electric*, 102–103.

28. Brock, *Charlatan*, 20.

29. Whorton, *Inner Hygiene*, 154.

30. John H. Girdner, "Healing by Electricity," *Munsey's Magazine*, 29, Apr 1903, 85.

31. Gant, *Constipation and Intestinal Obstruction*, 295.

32. Peña, *The Body Electric*, 143.

33. Green, *Fit for America*, 74.

34. Summers, *Bound to Please*, 91.

35. Advertisement in the *Illustrated London News*, Apr 10, 1880.

36. Walsh, *Cures*, 167–168.

37. Holbrook, *The Golden Age of Quackery*, 258.

38. Green, *Fit for America*, 174.

39. Walsh, *Cures*, 169–170.

40. U.S. Patent No. 1,190,831.

41. Holbrook, *The Golden Age of Quackery*, 36.

42. McCoy, *Quack*, 64.

43. Advertising for Dr. Scott's Electric Hairbrush in *The Graphic*, Oct 13, 1883.

44. *The Pathfinder*, 29, Feb 18, 1922, 11.

45. Cramp, *Nostrums and Quackery*, 220.

46. *Electreat Relieves Pain*. Peoria, Illinois: Electreat Manufacturing Co., 1919.

47. McCoy, *Quack*, 51.

48. Gardner, *Fads and Fallacies in the Name of Science*, 210–211.

Chapter Seven

1. George M. Beard, "Neurasthenia, or Nervous Exhaustion," *Boston Medical and Surgical Journal*, III, 1869, 217. For further details, see also the books by Beard listed in the bibliography.

2. Haller and Haller, *The Physician and Sexuality in Victorian America*, 6–7.

3. Peña, *The Body Electric*, 4.

4. Haller and Haller, *The Physician and Sexuality in Victorian America*, 15.

5. Beard and Rockwell, *Sexual Neurasthenia*, 75.

6. Marlin Gardner and Benjamin H. Aylworth, *The Domestic Physician and Family*

Assistant (Cooperstown: H&E Phinney, 1836), 115–116.

7. Peña, *The Body Electric*, 26.

8. For a further explanation and a more detailed understanding of the confusion between hysteria, chlorosis, and neurasthenia and their changing meanings and treatments, see Veith, *Hysteria* (1965); Haller and Haller, *The Physician and Sexuality in Victorian America* (1974); Maines, *The Technology of Orgasm* (1999), 21–42; and Laurinda S. Dixon, "Some Penetrating Insights," *Art Journal*, Fall, 1993.

9. Haller and Haller, *The Physician and Sexuality in Victorian America*, 12–13.

10. Armstrong and Armstrong, *The Great American Medicine Show*, 218.

11. Haller and Haller, *The Physician and Sexuality in Victorian America*, 11, 23.

12. McLaren, *Impotence*, 139.

13. Beard and Rockwell, *Sexual Neurasthenia*, 249.

14. McLaren, *Impotence*, 143. In the modern world, electrical stimulation of the rectum is commonly used on bulls and stallions to produce sperm for artificial insemination. In 1984, doctors with the Veteran's Administration tried to gather sperm with similar techniques from veterans with spinal cord injuries in order that they might father children. Warner, Harold, et al.: "Electrostimulation of Erection and Ejaculation and Collection of Semen in Spinal Cord Injured Humans," *Journal of Rehabilitation Research and Development*, 23 (3), 1986, 21–31.

15. Beard: *Sexual Neurasthenia*, 250.

16. Snow, *Mechanical Vibration and Its Therapeutic Application*, 21–24.

17. Wroebel, *Pseudo-Science and Society in Nineteenth-Century America*, 55.

18. Wroebel, *Pseudo-Science and Society in Nineteenth-Century America*, 60.

19. Maines, *The Technology of Orgasm*, 33.

Chapter Eight

1. Armstrong and Armstrong, *The Great American Medicine Show*, 190.

2. Holbrook, *The Golden Age of Quackery*, 36.

3. Armstrong and Armstrong, *The Great American Medicine Show*, 191.

4. Green, *Fit for America*, 75.

5. Approximately the same buying power today as $600.

6. Peña, *The Body Electric*, 110.

7. Approximately $130 in today's buying power.

8. Medical Battery Company advertising in *Illustrated London News*, Apr 10, 1880.

9. Wroebel, *Pseudo-Science and Society in Nineteenth-Century America*, 59.

10. Sears, Roebuck & Co. Catalog No. 110, Fall 1900, 38.

11. Approximately $540 in today's buying power.

12. Sears, Roebuck & Co. Catalog No. 110, Fall 1900, 38.

13. *Catalog of the Owen's Belts and Appliances*, 1890.

14. Wroebel, *Pseudo-Science and Society in Nineteenth-Century America*, 54.

15. Pulvermacher's Galvanic Company brochure, *The Only Rational Means for Self-Cure*.

16. Holbrook, *The Golden Age of Quackery*, 140.

17. Peña, *The Body Electric*, 1, 128.

18. George J. Duraind, *Gaylord Wilshire and His Amazing Discovery* (Los Angeles: Iona Company, 1927), 9.

19. I-ON-A-CO advertising in *Liberty*, Feb 26, 1927.

20. Holbrook, *The Golden Age of Quackery*, 143.

21. McCoy, *Quack*, 37.

22. Holbrook, *The Golden Age of Quackery*, 140.

23. Lisa Rosner, *The Technological Fix: How People Use Technology to Create and Solve Problems* (London: Taylor & Francis: 2004), 33.

24. Peña, *The Body Electric*, 132.

25. Holbrook, *The Golden Age of Quackery*, 141.

26. *Detroit Free Press*, Feb 17, 1929.

27. McCoy, *Quack*, 40–41.

28. Holbrook, *The Golden Age of Quackery*, 37.

29. Cramp, *Nostrums and Quackery*, 244–245.

30. Peña, *The Body Electric*, 123.

31. Cramp, *Nostrums and Quackery*, 245.

32. The Gibson Girl appeared in a series of sketches created by Charles Dana Gibson for *Life* magazine in 1887, and which lasted until about 1910. Refined, graceful, and stately, she was supposed to represent the ideal image of the American young woman.

33. Cramp, *Nostrums and Quackery*, 255–257.

34. Holbrook, *The Golden Age of Quackery*, 123–126.

35. *The Searchlight* (*Journal of Oxypathy*), 1 (2), Dec 1909.

36. McCoy, *Quack*, 47.

37. Gardner, *Fads and Fallacies in the Name of Science*, 104–105.

38. F.A. Archdale, *Elementary Radiesthesia and the Use of the Pendulum* (Pomeroy, WA: Health Research, 1961), 1.

39. Simon A. Senzon, "The Chiropractic Vertebral Subluxation Part 4: New Perspectives and Theorists From 1916 to 1927," *Journal of Chiropractic Humanities*, 25, Dec 2018, 52–66.

40. B.J. Palmer Chiropractic Clinic. "The electroencephaloneuromentimpograph: and its use in the B.J. Palmer Chiropractic Clinic." Davenport, IA: The Clinic, 1937.

41. MacIvor and LaForest, *Vibrations*, 74.

42. Kang and Pedersen, *Quackery*, 306–311.

43. Holbrook, *The Golden Age of Quackery*, 132–133.

44. Gardner, *Fads and Fallacies in the Name of Science*, 207.

45. Kang and Pedersen, *Quackery*, 309–310.

46. McCoy, *Quack*, 80.

47. Gardner, *Fads and Fallacies in the Name of Science*, 206.

48. Armstrong and Armstrong, *The Great American Medicine Show*, 194.

49. Armstrong and Armstrong, *The Great American Medicine Show*, 194.

50. Gardner, *Fads and Fallacies in the Name of Science*, 339.

51. David V. Tansley, *Radionics—Interface with the Ether-Fields* (Holsworthy, England: Health Science Press, 2011), xv.

52. McCoy, *Quack*, 117–118.

53. Gardner, *Fads and Fallacies in the Name of Science*, 209.

54. Stephen Barrett, "The Toftness Radiation Detector Is a Bogus Device," *Chirobase*, May 17, 2017.

55. Editorial Staff, "Abrams-like Devices Are Toftness-like Devices and Rubbing Plates," *Dynamic Chiropractic*, 9 (14), Jul 5, 1991.

56. McCoy, *Quack*, 121.

57. U.S. Patent No. 2,028,378; see also note #6 for Chapter 5 concerning the ether.

58. McCoy, *Quack*, 122.

59. For example, John Wilkes, *Radionics: Theory and Practice*. London: Herbert Jenkins, 1960.

60. MacIvor and LaForest, *Vibrations*, 76.

61. MacIvor and LaForest, *Vibrations*, 72.

62. MacIvor and LaForest, *Vibrations*, 75.

63. MacIvor and LaForest, *Vibrations*, 86–87.

64. McCoy, *Quack*, 92–93.

Chapter Nine

1. Terry W. Mangan, *Colorado on Glass: Colorado's First Half Century As Seen by the Camera* (Silverton, CO: Sundance, 1975), 304.

2. Cramp, *Nostrums and Quackery: Volume II*, 690–693.

3. The velocipede was the name for an early type of bicycle.

4. Hart-Davis, *What the Victorians Did for Us*, 135.

5. Whorton, *Inner Hygiene*, 185–186.

6. Peña, *The Body Electric*, 84–85.

7. Gant, *Constipation and Intestinal Obstruction*, 221, 280.

8. Maines, *The Technology of Orgasm*, 4.

9. Maines, *The Technology of Orgasm*, 11.

10. The Battle Creek Sanitarium in Michigan was one of the largest sanitariums in the country in the late 1800s and Dr. Kellogg was the superintendent who developed many innovative treatments. For more on Kellogg and his machinery see Chapter 14 in Agnew, *Healing Waters* or one of the Kellogg books listed in the bibliography. For a lighter view of Kellogg and the sanitarium, and the absurd side of spa therapy, the curious might enjoy the satirical motion picture *The Road to Wellville* (1994), with Anthony Hopkins as Kellogg.

11. Peña, *The Body Electric*, 79.

12. McCoy, *Quack*, 30.

13. McCoy, *Quack*, 29.

14. Maines, *The Technology of Orgasm*, 4.

15. Maines, *The Technology of Orgasm*, 10.

16. Belofsky, *Strange Medicine*, 125.

17. Helen King, "Galen and the widow. Towards a history of therapeutic masturbation in ancient gynecology," *EuGeStA:*

Journal on Gender Studies in Antiquity, 1, 2011, 205–235.

18. Hallie Lieberman and Eric Schatzberg, "A Failure of Academic Quality Control: The Technology of Orgasm," *Journal of Positive Sexuality*, 4 (2), Aug 2018, 24–47.

19. Granville, Mortimer J. *Nerve-Vibration and Excitation as Agents in the Treatment of Functional Disorder and Organic Disease*. (London: J & A Churchill, 1883) 57.

20. See Maines, *The Technology of Orgasm*; see also: Rachel Maines, "Socially camouflaged technologies: the case of the electromechanical vibrator," *IEEE Technology and Society Magazine*, 8 (2), Jun 1989.

21. Margolis, *The Intimate History of the Orgasm*, 245.

22. Maines, *The Technology of Orgasm*, 76–81.

23. Belofsky, *Strange Medicine*, 124.

24. Maines, *The Technology of Orgasm*, 14–15.

25. Kang and Pedersen, *Quackery*, 249.

26. More specific examples are referenced in Note 70 for Chapter 1 in Maines, *The Technology of Orgasm*, 135.

27. *American Magazine* 75, 7, 1913, 127.

28. Maines, *The Technology of Orgasm*, 20.

29. Green, *Fit for America*, 145.

30. Bertha Harmer and Virginia Henderson, *Textbook of the Principles and Practice of Nursing* (New York: Macmillan, 1960), 663–665.

31. Allied Merke advertising in *The Outlook*, Mar 21, 1923, 509.

32. Brock, *Charlatan*, photo section.

33. Allied Merke advertising in *Popular Mechanics*, May 1923, 21.

34. Haller and Haller, *The Physician and Sexuality in Victorian America*, 150.

35. Oneill, *Unmentionable*, 130–131.

36. Summers, *Bound to Please*, 88.

37. Whorton, *Crusaders for Fitness*, 101.

38. Haller and Haller, *The Physician and Sexuality in Victorian America*, 150.

39. Summers, *Bound to Please*, 88.

40. Kunzle, *Fashion and Fetishism*, 119.

41. Ewing, *Underwear*, 52.

42. Kunzle, *Fashion and Fetishism*, 119.

43. Ewing, *Underwear*, 51–52.

44. Green, *Fit for America*, 92.

45. Alice Stockham, *Tokology: A Book for Every Woman* (London: L.N. Fowler, 1900), 31.

46. Summers, *Bound to Please*, 112.

47. Haller and Haller, *The Physician and Sexuality in Victorian America*, 147.

48. Orson Fowler, *Tight-Lacing, Founded on Physiology and Phrenology; or, the Evils Inflicted on Mind and Body by Compressing the Organs of Animal Life, and Thereby Retarding and Enfeebling the Vital Functions* (New York: O.S. & L.N. Fowler, 1842), 48.

49. Green, *The Light of the Home*, 122–124.

50. Kunzle, *Fashion and Fetishism*, 137.

51. James R. Petersen, *The Century of Sex* (New York: Grove Press, 1999), 63.

52. *Mademoiselle*, Mar 1961.

53. Deutsch, *The New Nuts Among the Berries*, 205–206.

54. Food and Drug Administration, *Notices of Judgment Collection. Drugs and Devices, 1940–1963*. Washington, D.C. Case No. 6029.

Chapter Ten

1. Whorton, *Inner Hygiene*, xii.

2. Susan E. Cayleff, *Wash and Be Healed: The Water-Cure Movement and Women's Health* (Philadelphia: Temple University Press, 1987), 43.

3. Whorton, *Inner Hygiene*, xi.

4. Russell, *Colonic Irrigation*, 2–3.

5. Whorton, *Inner Hygiene*, 22.

6. Kellogg, *The Battle Creek Sanitarium System*, 13.

7. Whorton, *Inner Hygiene*, 146–147.

8. Kellogg, *Colon Hygiene*, 294.

9. Kellogg, *Colon Hygiene*, 292–293.

10. Gant, *Constipation and Intestinal Obstruction*, 281.

11. Gant, *Constipation and Intestinal Obstruction*, 515–516.

12. Charles D. Aaron, *Diseases of the Digestive Organs: With Special Reference to Their Diagnosis* (Philadelphia: Lea & Febiger, 1921), 229.

13. Whorton, *Inner Hygiene*, 153.

14. Snow, *Mechanical Vibration and Its Therapeutic Application*, 237–238.

15. Gant, *Constipation and Intestinal Obstruction*, 282.

16. Gant, *Constipation and Intestinal Obstruction*, 291.

17. Gant, *Constipation and Intestinal Obstruction*, 284–292.

18. Charles D. Aaron, *Diseases of the Digestive Organs: With Special Reference*

to Their Diagnosis (Philadelphia: Lea & Febiger, 1921), 231.

19. William W. Lieberman, "The Enema," *The Review of Gastroenterology*, 13 (3), 1946, 215–229.

20. Whorton, *Crusaders for Fitness*, 218.

21. Whorton, *Inner Hygiene*, 24.

22. Whorton, *Crusaders for Fitness*, 217.

23. Metchnikoff, *The Prolongation of Life*, 71.

24. Whorton, *Inner Hygiene*, 57–58.

25. William Arbuthnot Lane, "The Sewage System of the Human Body," *American Medicine*, 29, 1923, 267–272.

26. T. Coraghessan Boyle, *The Road to Wellville* (New York: Penguin, 1993), 253.

27. Whorton, *Inner Hygiene*, 66.

28. Gant, *Constipation and Intestinal Obstruction*, 43.

29. Jamison, *Intestinal Irrigation*, 6.

30. Russell, *Colonic Irrigation*, 3.

31. Whorton, *Crusaders for Fitness*, 216–217.

32. Gant, *Constipation and Intestinal Obstruction*, 277.

33. Irina Matveikova, *Digestive Intelligence* (Forres, Scotland: Findhorn Press, 2016), 102.

34. Whorton, *Inner Hygiene*, 121.

35. Russell, *Colonic Irrigation*, 89.

36. Jamison, Alcinous. *Intestinal Irrigation: or Why, How, and When to Flush the Colon* (New York: published by the author, 1914), 1.

37. Russell, *Colonic Irrigation*, 20.

38. GB Patent No. 323,834A.

39. Russell, *Colonic Irrigation*, 100–101.

40. Honsaker Lavagatory, U.S. Patent No. 1,818,978.

41. Russell, *Colonic Irrigation*, 71.

42. Russell, *Colonic Irrigation*, 147. That is with nine or ten patients per day, assuming a five-day work week.

43. Whorton, *Inner Hygiene*, 136.

44. Russell, *Colonic Irrigation*, 111.

45. Alexander G. Gibson, "The Use of the Plombières Douche," *Proceedings of the Royal Society of Medicine* (Section of Balneology and Climatology), May 5, 1923, 22–23. There is currently some controversial hypothetical thinking that stimulation of the large intestine through colonic irrigation may stimulate the release of endorphins in the abdomen, which may help to contribute to this feeling of well-being; however, no proof of this has been established.

46. Whorton, *Inner Hygiene*, 128.

47. In reality, the device was invented and patented in 1903 by Henry M. Guild. U.S. Patents No. 730,822 and No. 757,654 were merely assigned to Tyrrell's Hygienic Institute. A very similar device had actually been patented previously in 1894 by Joseph Lalonde.

48. Tyrrell, *The Royal Road to Health*, 66. This name was as simplistic as the I-ON-A-CO name used by Gaylord Wilshire for the electric collar described in Chapter 8.

49. Whorton, *Inner Hygiene*, 129–130.

50. Whorton, *Inner Hygiene*, 133–134.

51. Gant, *Constipation and Intestinal Obstruction*, 237.

52. Alcinous B. Jamison, *Intestinal Ills* (New York: Knickerbocker Press, 1901), 207.

53. Alcinous B. Jamison, *Intestinal Irrigation* (New York: published by the author, 1901), 100.

54. Whorton, *Inner Hygiene*, 127.

55. Oneill, *Unmentionable*, 178–179.

Chapter Eleven

1. McCoy, *Quack*, 158.

2. Souter, *The Doctor's Bag*, 294.

3. Watkins, *A Manual of Electrotherapy*, 13.

4. Joseph B. DeLee and Mabel C. Carmon, *Obstetrics for Nurses* (Philadelphia: W.B. Saunders, 1939), 436.

5. U.S. Patent No. 2,328,640.

6. Burdick, *Infra-Red Therapy*, 17, 21, 30, 31.

7. Vestvold, *The Naturopath and Herald of Health* (1935), 191; U.S. Patent No. 1,951,569.

8. Food and Drug Administration, *Notices of Judgment Collection. Drugs and Devices, 1940–1963*. Washington, D.C. Case No. 2987.

9. Kang and Pedersen, *Quackery*, 301.

10. Renulife Electric Company, *Renulife Violet Ray Manual* (Detroit: Renulife Electric Company, 1919), 5.

11. These were not the same as today's Violet Wand devices that are used for sexual stimulation, particularly in the S&M community, by applying electricity to the erogenous zones.

12. Peña, *The Body Electric*, 126.

13. Peña, *The Body Electric*, 121, 125.

14. Vi-Rex advertising in *Argosy All-Story Weekly*, Sep 1921, and *Science and Invention*, Feb 1925.

15. *Renulife Violet Ray Manual*, 1919.

16. Gardner, *Fads and Fallacies in the Name of Science*, 212–213.

17. McCoy, *Quack*, 119.

18. For comparison, most home reading lamps use 60, 75, or 100 watt lightbulbs.

19. Gardner, *Fads and Fallacies in the Name of Science*, 211, 339–340; also Proceedings from Court Action, State of Illinois versus William M. Estep and Dora Estep, Feb 11, 1952.

20. Rolls, *Diseased, Douched and Doctored*, 40–41.

21. McCoy, *Quack*, 67–68.

22. Walsh, *Cures*, 172–173.

23. Augustus J. Pleasanton. *The Influence Of The Blue Ray Of The Sunlight And Of The Blue Colour Of The Sky: In developing animal and vegetable life; in arresting disease, and in restoring health in acute and chronic disorders to human and domestic animals.* Philadelphia: Claxton, Remsen & Haffelfinger, 1877.

24. *The Gazette*, Colorado Springs, CO, Dec 11, 2008.

Chapter Twelve

1. Steinbach, *Women in England 1760–1914*, 109.

2. Haller and Haller, *The Physician and Sexuality in Victorian America*, x–xi.

3. Steinbach, *Women in England 1760–1914*, 108.

4. McLaren, *Impotence*, xii.

5. McLaren, *Impotence*, 85–86.

6. McLaren, *Impotence*, 182.

7. Haller and Haller, *The Physician and Sexuality in Victorian America*, 233.

8. Holbrook, *The Golden Age of Quackery*, 251.

9. McLaren, *Impotence*, 183.

10. E. Schubert and M. Zolotnitsky, "Sklerator: A Device for the Treatment of Male Impotence by Mechanical Means," *Zeitschrift für Urologie*, 16, Feb 1922, 83.

11. Brock, *Charlatan*, 184.

12. McCoy, *Quack*, 223.

13. Holbrook, *The Golden Age of Quackery*, 73.

14. Cramp, *Nostrums and Quackery*, 259.

15. Kang and Pedersen, *Quackery*, 207.

16. Belofsky, *Strange Medicine*, 123.

17. Peña, *The Body Electric*, 151.

18. McLaren, *Impotence*, 86.

19. McLaren, *Impotence*, xi.

20. Frederick Hollick, *A Popular Treatise on Venereal Diseases, in All Their Forms. Embracing Their History, and Probable Origin; Their Consequences, Both to Individuals and to Society; and the Best Modes of Treating Them* (New York: 1852), 69.

21. Margolis, *The Intimate History of the Orgasm*, 287.

22. McCoy, *Quack*, 61.

23. Reich, *The Function of the Orgasm*, 383–385.

24. Gardner, *Fads and Fallacies in the Name of Science*, 251–253.

25. Gardner, *Fads and Fallacies in the Name of Science*, 256.

26. McCoy, *Quack*, 154.

27. Gardner, *Fads and Fallacies in the Name of Science*, 344.

28. Rolls, *Diseased, Douched and Doctored*, 170.

29. The phlogiston theory was put forward in the 1660s in an attempt to explain combustion, but was later found to be false. Phlogiston was a supposed substance that was contained in combustible materials and was released when they burned. De-phlogistonation was the process of releasing phlogiston into the air, where it was absorbed. Graham's ideas of linking this to health seems unclear.

30. £2 was equivalent to a skilled tradesman's wages for two days.

31. Gardner, *Fads and Fallacies in the Name of Science*, 244.

32. Porter, *Quacks*, 145.

33. Sutcliffe and Duin, *A History of Medicine*, 43. Again, it is difficult to value this amount because of time, inflation, and exchange rates, but this was probably worth about $4,000 in purchasing power today, a very large amount of money at the time. At the time this amount would purchase four horses, or was the wages of a skilled tradesman for about a year.

34. McLaren, *Impotence*, 187.

35. Kang and Pedersen, *Quackery*, 238–240.

36. Brock, *Charlatan*, 37.

37. McCoy, *Quack*, 223.

38. Peña, *The Body Electric*, 165.

39. Box labeling for Dr. Young's Ideal Self-Retaining Rectal Dilators.

40. Gant, *Constipation and Intestinal Obstruction*, 520.

41. "Pneumatic Dilator," *Herald of Health and Naturopath*, 1918, 23.

42. Kang and Pedersen, *Quackery*, 207.

43. Advertising for the Recto Rotor.

44. Peña, *The Body Electric*, 166–167.

45. U.S. Patent No. 1,279,111.

46. McCoy, *Quack*, 230.

47. Peña, *The Body Electric*, 167.

48. Peña, *The Body Electric*, 169.

Chapter Thirteen

1. Some of the first people to use uranium were pre-historic Native Americans who mined carnotite ore (the source of uranium, radium, and vanadium) to make yellow pigment to paint murals on the walls of desert cliffs in southern Utah. Later, Ute Indians used the same ore to make warpaint.

2. Half-life is the length of time required for the spontaneous disintegration of half the atoms in a sample of radioactive material. The half-life of radium is 1590 years.

3. Peña, *The Body Electric*, 191–192.

4. Rolls, *Diseased, Douched and Doctored*, 51.

5. Basil B. Creighton, "Manitou Springs," *Chicago Medical Recorder*, Sep 1915, 10–11.

6. Guy Hinsdale, *Hydrotherapy; A Work on Hydrotherapy in General, Its Application to Special Affectations, the Technic or Processes Employed, and the Use of Waters Internally* (Philadelphia: W.B. Saunders, 1910), 390–391.

7. Peña, *The Body Electric*, 195, 197.

8. Kang and Pedersen, *Quackery*, 48.

9. *Silver City Independent*, Jun 14, 1921.

10. Rolls, *Diseased, Douched and Doctored*, 51.

11. Kang and Pedersen, *Quackery*, 50.

12. Advertising for treatment of the sex glands reproduced in McCoy, *Quack*, 112.

At the time "spicy," "snappy," and "peppy" were well-known code words for sexy.

13. Kang and Pedersen, *Quackery*, 50.

14. Radioactive emissions are of three types (alpha, beta, and gamma), though not all radioactive substances give off all three. Alpha radiation consists of an emitted nucleus of helium (two protons, two neutrons). Beta radiation consists of electrons moving at high speed. Both of these are relatively harmless to humans, though beta radiation can penetrate living tissue, causing genetic damage, and concentrated beams of electrons are used for cancer therapy. However, the most penetrating and damaging of the three types is gamma radiation, which consists of powerful electromagnetic energy, somewhat like X-rays, which creates serious biological damage to human cells and tissue.

15. McCoy, *Quack*, 105.

16. Thoron is a radioactive isotope of radon that is formed as a decay byproduct of the decomposition of thorium. It has a half-life of less than a minute.

17. Jim Mahaffey, *Atomic Accidents: A History of Nuclear Meltdowns and Disasters*. New York: Pegasus Books, 2014.

18. Peña, *The Body Electric*, 198–199.

19. Kang and Pedersen, *Quackery*, 45.

20. The author was personally acquainted with two men who owned and operated a medical X-ray facility in the 1960s. They told him that when they first started the business, they X-rayed each other up and down over and over again to in order to gain practice on their machine. When they later came to understand the dangers involved, they of course regretted the practice.

21. Belofsky, *Strange Medicine*, 167.

22. Council A. Nedd, "When the Solution was the Problem: A Brief History of the Shoe Fluoroscope," *American Journal of Roentgenology*, 158 (6), 1992, 1270.

Bibliography

Agnew, Jeremy. *Healing Waters: A History of Victorian Spas*. Jefferson, NC: McFarland, 2019.

Agnew, Jeremy. *Medicine in the Old West: A History 1850–1900*. Jefferson, NC: McFarland, 2010.

Anderson, Ann. *Snake Oil, Hustlers and Hambones: The American Medicine Show*. Jefferson, NC: McFarland, 2000.

Armstrong, David, and Elizabeth M. Armstrong. *The Great American Medicine Show*. New York: Prentice-Hall, 1991.

Beard, George M. *American Nervousness: Its Causes and Consequences*. New York: G.P. Putnam's Sons, 1881.

Beard, George M. *A Practical Treatise on Nervous Exhaustion (Neurasthenia): Its Symptoms, Nature, Sequences, Treatment*. New York: E.B. Treat, 1894.

Beard, George M., and Alphonso D. Rockwell. *A Practical Treatise on the Medical and Surgical Uses of Electricity*. New York: William Wood, 1871.

Beard, George M., and Alphonso D. Rockwell. *Sexual Neurasthenia [Nervous Exhaustion]: Its Hygiene, Causes, Symptoms and Treatment*. New York: E.B. Treat, 1900.

Belofsky, Nathan. *Strange Medicine: A Shocking History of Real Medical Practices Through the Ages*. New York: Perigee/Penguin, 2013.

Brock, Pope. *Charlatan: America's Most Dangerous Huckster, the Man Who Pursued Him, and the Age of Flimflam*. New York: Crown Publishers, 2008.

Burdick, Frederick F. *Infra-Red Therapy*. Milton, WI: Burdick Research Laboratories, 1923.

Child, Lydia M. *The Family Nurse: or Companion of the American Frugal Housewife*. Boston: Charles J. Hendee, 1837.

Coolidge, Frederick L. *Statistics*. London: Sage Publications, 2000.

Cramp, Arthur J. *Nostrums and Quackery: Volume II*. Chicago: American Medical Association, 1921.

Cramp, Arthur J. (ed). *Nostrums and Quackery*. (Collected and edited from Vols I, II, III). Chicago: American Medical Association, 1936.

Dary, David. *Frontier Medicine: From the Atlantic to the Pacific, 1492–1941*. New York: Alfred A. Knopf, 2008.

Deutsch, Ronald M. *The New Nuts Among the Berries*. Palo Alto: Bull Publishing, 1977.

Ewing, Elizabeth. *Underwear: A History*. New York: Theater Arts Books, 1972.

Fowler, Orson S., and Lorenzo N. Fowler. *The Illustrated Self-Instructor in Phrenology and Physiology*. New York: Fowler and Wells, 1857.

Gant, Samuel G. *Constipation and Intestinal Obstruction*. Philadelphia: W.B. Saunders, 1909.

Gardner, Martin. *Fads and Fallacies in the Name of Science*. New York: Dover, 1957.

Green, Harvey. *Fit for America: Health, Fitness, Sport and American Society*. New York: Pantheon Books, 1986.

Green, Harvey. *The Light of the Home*. New York: Pantheon Books, 1983.

Haller, John S., and Robin M. Haller. *The Physician and Sexuality in Victorian America*. Urbana: University of Illinois Press, 1974.

Hart-Davis, Adam. *What the Victorians Did for Us*. London: Headline Book Publishing, 2001.

Holbrook, Stewart H. *The Golden Age of Quackery*. New York: Macmillan, 1959.

Janik, Erika. *Marketplace of the Marvelous. The Strange Origins of Modern Medicine*. Boston: Beacon Press, 2014.

Kang, Lydia, and Nate Pedersen. *Quackery: A Brief History of the Worst Ways to Cure Everything*. New York: Workman Publishing, 2017.

Kellogg, John H. *Autointoxication or Intestinal Toxemia*. Battle Creek, MI: Modern Medicine Publishing, 1919.

Kellogg, John H. *The Battle Creek Sanitarium System: History, Organization, Methods*. Battle Creek, (MI: no publisher), 1908.

Kellogg, John H. *Colon Hygiene*. Battle Creek, MI: Good Health Publishing, 1915.

Kunzle, David. *Fashion and Fetishism: Corsets, Tight-Lacing and Other Forms of Body-Sculpture*. Phoenix Mill, UK: Sutton Publishing, 2004.

MacIvor, Virginia, and Sandra LaForest. *Vibrations: Healing Through Color Homeopathy and Radionics*. York Beach, ME: Samuel Weiser, 1979.

Maines, Rachel P. *The Technology of Orgasm*. Baltimore: Johns Hopkins University Press, 1999.

Margolis, Jonathan. *O: The Intimate History of the Orgasm*. New York: Grove Press, 2004.

McCoy, Bob. *Quack: Tales of Medical Fraud from the Museum of Questionable Medical Devices*. Santa Monica: Santa Monica Press, 2000.

McLaren, Angus. *Impotence: A Cultural History*. Chicago: University of Chicago Press, 2007.

Metchnikoff, Élie. *The Prolongation of Life*. New York: G.P. Putnam's Sons, 1908.

Morris, Thomas. *The Mystery of the Exploding Teeth (And Other Curiosities from the World of Medicine)*. New York: Dutton, 2018.

Oneill, Therese. *Unmentionable: The Victorian Lady's Guide to Sex, Marriage and Manners*. New York: Little Brown, 2016.

Parker, Steve. *Medicine: The Definitive Illustrated History*. New York: Penguin Random House, 2016.

Peña, Carolyn T. de la. *The Body Electric: How Strange Machines Built the Modern America*. New York: New York University Press, 2003.

Porter, Roy. *The Greatest Benefit to Mankind: A Medical History of Humanity*. New York: W.W. Norton, 1997.

Porter, Roy. *Quacks: Fakers and Charlatans in English Medicine*. Stroud, UK: Tempus Publishing, 2001.

Reich, Wilhelm. *The Function of the Orgasm: Sex-Economic Problems of Biological Energy*. New York: Farrar, Straus and Giroux, 1973.

Rolls, Roger. *Diseased, Douched and Doctored: Thermal Springs, Spa Doctors and Rheumatic Diseases*. London: London Publishing Partnership, 2012.

Rumsey, Deborah J. *Statistics for Dummies*. Hoboken, NJ: Wiley, 2011.

Russell, William Kerr. *Colonic Irrigation*. Edinburgh: E&S Livingstone, 1932.

Rutkow, Ira. *Seeking the Cure: A History of Medicine in America*. New York: Scribner's, 2010.

Snow, Mary L. *Mechanical Vibration and Its Therapeutic Application*. New York: Scientific Author Publishing, 1904.

Souter, Keith. *The Doctor's Bag: Medicine and Surgery of Yesteryear*. No city: Sundown Press, 2015.

Steele, Volney. *Bleed, Blister and Purge: A History of Medicine on the American Frontier.* Missoula: Mountain Press Publishing, 2005.

Steinbach, Susie. *Women in England 1760–1914: A Social History.* London: Weidenfeld & Nicolson, 2004.

Summers, Leigh. *Bound to Please: A History of the Victorian Corset.* Oxford, UK: Berg, 2001.

Sutcliffe, Jenny, and Nancy Duin. *A History of Medicine.* London: Morgan Samuel Editions, 1992.

Thompson, Damian. *Counterknowledge.* New York: W.W. Norton, 2008.

Toledo-Pereyra, Luis H. *A History of American Medicine from the Colonial Period to the Early Twentieth Century.* Lewiston, ME: Edward Mellen Press, 2006.

Tyrrell, Charles A. *The Royal Road to Health: or the Secret of Health Without Drugs.* New York: Tyrrell's Hygenic Institute, 1917.

Veith, Ilza. *Hysteria: The History of a Disease.* Chicago: University of Chicago Press, 1965.

Walsh, James J. *Cures: The Story of the Cures That Fail.* New York: D. Appleton, 1923.

Warren, David J. *Old Medical and Dental Instruments.* Princes Risborough, UK: Shire Publications, 1994.

Watkins, Arthur L. *A Manual of Electrotherapy.* New York: Lea & Febiger, 1958.

Whorton, James C. *Crusaders for Fitness: The History of American Health Reformers.* Princeton, NJ: Princeton University Press, 1982.

Whorton, James C. *Inner Hygiene: Constipation and the Pursuit of Health in Modern Society.* New York: Oxford University Press, 2000.

Whorton, James C. *Nature Cures: The History of Alternative Medicine in America.* New York: Oxford University Press, 2002.

Wroebel, Arthur. *Pseudo-Science and Society in Nineteenth-Century America.* Lexington: University Press of Kentucky, 1987.

Index

Numbers in **_bold italics_** refer to pages with illustrations

275